PRAISE FOR *KAMI*

M000073593

"What a delightful fusion of Yoga and Christianity! Fresh and funny, irreverently reverent, wise and empowering. *Kamikaze Yogi* is an accessible guide to reclaiming our inherent divinity and saying a full-bodied *yes* to life."

MIRABAI STARR, AUTHOR OF *GOD OF LOVE* AND *WILD MERCY*

"This book, named in honor of a loved one lost too early to cancer, is written for those who yearn to befriend their true Self, which exists below ego. Leaning into Christian mysticism while drawing from Judaism, Hindu and Buddhist traditions, this book is simultaneously an interactive workbook and a memoir/spiritual journey. Perhaps it is better to say that Anita's spiritual journey, expressed with brutal honesty and tender vulnerability, is translated into a roadmap for others to follow, if they so choose. Readers are taken on a meandering, boundary-breaking pilgrimage, best traveled when presumptions and preconceived notions are checked at the door. Choose the sacred, when so many are scared; the repositioning of one letter, the reading of this book, may result in a profound, life-giving, shift."

REBECCA BRYAN, CONSULTANT AND NURSE

"This book is an invitation that beckons healing. As a pastor and chaplain, I know we all need this "comfy chair". Anita writes to the reader as though we are sitting in her home office or yoga studio doing this healing work. She asks deep, meaningful questions, while sharing her own vulnerable places and healing. She takes us on a voyage of the particularities of "mind/body yoking"—how we can honor the places in us that cannot be divided; the ones Jesus refers to. I found the following sentence almost musical, "Though every cell has incredible intelligence, the heart is the center of our physical and spiritual life, an organ of ethereal perception." I will think of and hear my church organ differently. How beautiful a global congregation is that joins virtually with hearts and minds. Read this book! It is a gift during such a trying time. Breathe and unclench those jaws and drop your shoulders!"

MONICA BANKS

"Reading *Kamikaze Yogi* feels like a long, restorative chat with a trusted, straight-talking friend who loves you too much to let you stay imprisoned within the confines of your own closed mind. What a gift this book is! Anita Grace Brown empowers us to leave behind the grave clothes of our preconceptions about God, mysticism, our fellow humans, and even ourselves. Don't miss this book! There is life and light for every single one of us in these pages."

JASON ELAM, HOST, THE MESSY SPIRITUALITY PODCAST

"*Kamikaze Yogi* is a provocative invitation to an embodied, East-meets-West path to awakening that focuses on redemption. Her own story of healing gives hope through an informative look at the chakra systems and a tutorial to everything yoga. This delightful book will take you on a journey of transformation that is helpful."

KARL FOREHAND, AUTHOR OF *APPARENT FAITH* AND *THE TEA SHOP*, AND CREATOR OF "THE DESERT SANCTUARY"

"Riveting and heartfelt, Anita invites all on a journey of self-discovery—a spiritual one in which Jesus is indeed the way, the truth, and the life; where yoga and mindfulness are pathways to experiencing the fullness of the abundant life God promises to every believer. In this masterpiece, Anita's captivating stories liberate the mind while inviting spirit to dance along and engage in activities that bring healing to the heart. Your inner child will thank you (this is the incarnation!) as peace saturates your soul and warmly embraces you in the here and now. Come, with open hearts, to receive, as Anita challenges each of us to embrace the sacred-body, soul, and spirit unified and steeped in divine love."

SIO WEDDERBURN, URBAN PROMISE INTERNATIONAL

"I can feel the genuine, warm place in the author's heart. *Kamikaze Yogi* is a great, insightful read...graceful!"

DONTE MOORE, PASTOR/FOUNDER BREAKTHROUGH MINISTRIES

KAMIKAZE YOGI

Christ, Yoga, and the Courage to Emerge

Anita Grace Brown

First Edition

Cover design and layout by Rafael Polendo (polendo.net)
Cover image courtesy of GraphicStock.com

ISBN 978-1-7348234-3-1

This volume is printed on acid free paper and meets ANSI Z39.48 standards.

Printed in the United States of America

Published by Shaia-Sophia House
An imprint of Quoir
San Antonio, Texas, USA

www.ShaiaSophiaHouse.com

Dedicated to the fragile child within
and the warrior who liberates her.

*"I saw the angel in the marble
and carved until I set him free."*

MICHELANGELO

ACKNOWLEDGMENTS

It takes a village to raise a child. It's the same for a book. My sincere gratitude to all those who have tutored me in every aspect of life, without your influence, this work would never have started, let alone received its final punctuation mark.

wholly thankful, Jesus
your aliveness compels the journey

profound love for my husband, Bob
you steadfastly hold the key to my kite; together we create electricity

tremendous pride for my son, Luke
wisdom beyond your years: you challenge me to dreaming and, oh joy!
how you help me remember to have fun

glorious wonderment over my daughter, Rebecca
fiercely, sincerely, + wholeheartedly independent, you influence me to be the best version of myself

dearest Mom
you dreamed me into this place + space

precious Oma,
every breeze on my cheek reminds me of the love which you gave as a second mom+ a sister

the miracles of twelve babies I nannied
blissfully sharing your wide-eyed innocence

magnanimous pastor Ben, and the holy COH family
as prayer warriors, your capacity of divine witnesses to the waves of
rising + falling is a living truth

dedicated friends: Liz, Renata, Heather, Cris, Mary Rita, Anne M,
Shikera
for walks + talks, texts + dreams—you pace my heart

spectacularly recognized and remembered, Kyle Teschko
you are the true meaning of kamikaze: divine wind

Sierra
my first soul beast, you are truly golden

Ryan K
you wisely told me the world needs me to bleed truth

Steve T & Mary L
my personal non-therapist therapists

Tippy
mentor extraordinaire, soulful sage

Bec
the gifter of Wild Goose Spirit

reaching out to the anonymous
thank you to the pastor who tried to exorcise my sexuality
for without Jesus redeeming of this violation,
I would not enjoy the wholeness of womanhood

literary blessings, Marie
the yang to my yin, lightly landing my words on earth

TABLE OF CONTENTS

PROLOGUE

It's a late May day
fierce winds as if March
no sign of the sun

I'm at my in-laws' beach house
to finish what God started
over two years ago:
this book

Last week
our 22-year-old daughter
graduated with high honors
on a full scholarship from Syracuse University
because of the pandemic
we could not celebrate her
capped + gowned in glorious joy—
nor celebrate the energy of life
the promise of future
in + with all the human doings
in her class of 2020

On this May day
I slightly resist
then go outside
to move my body
walk the dog
I pick up the pace
sprint for a block

Minutes later
on seeing a sign
displayed in a living room window
for someone named Bill
a new Rutgers graduate
I burst into tears
unable to touch the memory
that significant period of my life
when I graduated college
the first generation of my family
on American soil to do so

On this May day
I realize I have blocked out
much of my young adult life
too busy surviving
(before, then, after, + seemingly always)

Father forgive us
we know not what we do

We don't block + numb
because we want to
we don't intentionally
abandon our inner child
out of cruelty

On this May day
with fierce winds
purposefully stirring my inward sea
with a faceless Bill in the window

no caps-tossed-in-the-air at Syracuse
my own non-celebration folded away in a drawer of past
I weep openly

telling my 22-year-old
Self:

I haven't forgotten you
I am here
you are here
we are reunited

On this May day
the wind swirls 'round
my younger Self
the square on my calendar becomes emblazoned with TK
Talitha Koumi
the power of Aramaic words
spoken in scripture to a child
from the Son of Man's own mouth
a rebirth representing restoration + resurrection
as Jesus breathes new life
as those words reach me
on this May day
I boldly announce
Talitha Koumi

Arise little one
you were dormant
not dead

YOGA: MY STATEMENT ON CULTURAL APPROPRIATION

In this book, I write about practices that have their roots in the East. Yoga is such a practice. In scholarly study of mystics and practices, I offer a respectful bow to yoga's origins and acknowledge that it does not belong to the West, therefore it can never be fully understood by it. I believe that Yoga can be experienced, not owned. In all of my experiences, as I have come from a place of wonder, the invitations I have received to share in yoga have been benevolent and gracious.

I concede that certain aspects of sharing and inviting people to yoga could be interpreted as cultural appropriation.

My understanding, such as it is at this time, is that my practicing, and my inviting others to practice and celebrate movement, specifically yoga, is in reverence to yoga's origins. There is no intended corruption of origin, no commercial storefront in which agenda has pushed aside that respect, no geographical slight; nothing created or represented here in these pages has been done to exploit these sacred movements. I attempted to synthesize the most powerful aspects into seven basic tools. You can find much more detail on the book's YouTube channel as well as over 100 Jesus yoga episodes of my podcast "It's 5 o'clock Somewhere".

WELCOME, MAKE YOURSELF AT HOME. TAKE THE COMFY CHAIR

You are the cracked vessel from which the divine, fragrant elixir pours.

Are you smiling because you are such a phenomenon? A little surprised? Is there a little bit of doubt that you are the cracked vessel from which the divine, fragrant elixir pours? Yes, point that finger toward you and say, "Who, me?"

Yes, you.

Stay right where you are if peaceful wonder is already infusing your earthly reality. Just stand in your luminosity, bathe in the heavenliness of it all.

If you're still wondering, take some time to think about that. Is peace infusing your earthly reality?

YES   /   NO

Go ahead, circle one of those words (YES or NO). Do it with a pen or with your finger.

It's okay. Sure it might feel a little silly, but try it.

Whether you used your finger or a writing implement—or maybe you used an eye roll—however you did it, you just made a shape. I thank you for engaging right at the beginning with some somatic movement to consciously engage the body.

Do it again and let your vision follow the line you're making—be it in ink or just in the air over the word. That focus allowed you to be active and lose yourself in the thought of a shape. While 'you' were lost in that thought, even for a nanosecond, the 'you' who thinks you are in charge let go just a bit to be absorbed into the present moment. Each of us can recall those moments where we are free of the stress, free of the world, free of the critical voice in our heads. What are you doing? Maybe you are lost in a dance, making art or music, standing atop a mountain overlooking a grand vista?

How do you feel about the concept of peace within? Of the circle making? Let's do it again by circling the word or words that answer how you feel about that peace question:

CURIOUS   INTERESTED   INDIFFERENT   WEIRD

SUSPICIOUS   LOVED   SEEN   INVITED

We make shapes with our thoughts, words, and actions: stirring milk into coffee, walking the dog, teeth brushing, chin down (neck strained, shoulder sloped) staring at a screen, and kneeling before bed to pray.

As I flossed this morning, I reminded myself to tell you that the physical practice of yoga you're going to learn on these pages inaugurates a kind of cleansing to come because yoga is flossing for the body—and meditation is flossing for the mind. Claim your place here, right now. You belong.

About what I asked: is peace infusing your earthly reality?

If you live in that reality of experiencing peace beyond your ordinary understanding, then you, like me, are likely witnessing miracles first-hand. Your God is alive, for a new day has dawned, morning has broken through the darkness of night. Where grief had been-strangling your heart like a vice, there is freedom. Where fear's bony grip danced his somber moves, there is stillness in knowing the truth. Where shame once suffocated, snuffing out enchantment and delight, there is presence and mystery. Your new mind = you being a new creation. We were given one main command—embody the Love of God, for and with God.

Extend yourself and air-draw or pen-draw a happy face or sad face, or an expression between happy and sad. Simple, I know, but it's so much more. Really what you're doing is pausing from busy-ness, engaging in consciousness, and you're taking the first steps in interaction with my words. Now, take in a deep belly breath and sigh it out loudly (lots more on this later). Do it again, but even louder this time. Try buzzing your lips. Remember when you called that a zerbert?

If you are confused about whether a heavenly dimension is infusing your earthly reality, then likely it is not. If that's the case, taking the path of a kamikaze yogi will help you make a space to experience such a shift. The 'shift' is going to occur in your ordinary life as a deep experience in yourself as grounded and connected to nature, to soul, to breath, and so much more. These relationships, newly infused with Spirit, are going to save your mind from addiction to itself. Everywhere I go people agree, I am my own worst enemy.

When our 22-year-old daughter recently graduated with a degree in neuroscience, I asked her for help in explaining—based on her specialization and her knowing me—what shifted in my brain over the past eight years. I summarize her answer (and supplement it) this way: I speak in a more spiritual, poetic language than most, but all of this information can be understood by others from the perspective of the nervous system. All humans operate by using a portion of the brain in order to focus on the task at hand—things like holding a conversation or studying. If a person is distracted by memories, especially traumatic ones, that person struggles to live in the present.

As a form of protection and survival mechanism, the brain does not generally interrupt a person's life with flashbacks unless the person is suffering from extreme PTSD.

People dissociate, to a certain extent, from the energy of the body, the energy of the gut and heart brains, in order to work and enjoy life. Those who cannot function because of an overload of stored trauma ultimately seek help in the form of drugs (prescription or illegal) and/ or alcohol to numb the pain.

Maybe the ones who suffer from smaller, more typical traumas, have become so patterned in their conditioned thinking that they do not pursue healing in the present with somatic tools of mindful presence.

After eight years of daily centering prayer and yoga shapes, I discovered what it means to live in a state of prayer—in a state where I do not have to cease meditation. First, there was an uncovering of underlying survival physiology before my behavior and thinking evolved. Then, I discovered heaven on earth.

May my story inspire you to discover you are more resilient and wiser than you know.

Karma and Other Crap We Believe to Be the 'Be All/ End All'

You'll come to know me, a woman who once came at life with tense, closed fists, ready for a fight, now as one who arrives again and again from a wholly different place: softer, spacious, reconciled.

If karma is a natural law, and history repeats itself, if people don't really change, and the apple doesn't fall far from the tree, I shouldn't be writing this book. I should be trapped in a body-mind infused with the pain of my ancestors, coupled with decades of my own experiences of physical, sexual, and emotional trauma and abuse. I should be chronically ill, binge drinking, divorced, and unable to get free of Lexapro.

But for the grace of God go I. Jesus is beyond the law of karma; so are we.

I'll be honest here: for a long season, my yogic practices were not performed from pure motive. My reasons were clouded by not seeing myself clearly as beloved. Therefore, a little advice from hindsight: holding a vision of yourself as broken, damaged, or sinful, then doing yoga in order to 'fix' yourself is a 'no-no'.

Repeat after me, "I am loved completely just as I am."

I now come to my mat much more aware of being perfectly imperfect. My Spirit-filled heart is grounded in unshakeable virtue. Yes, always. I always begin and end with peace. As the first woman of deep faith in my family, I have a curious insight- it is much harder to go it alone- to not know where God is . I am the first one to wake up to the fact that the future was not written in my genes in permanent marker, that my prayers and actions, through grace, cause the wheels of karma to come to a screeching halt, that my great-grandchildren will benefit. An objective reality revealed in Christ has become my subjective reality through sanctification.

Can you believe that it is possible to be so filled with clarity? I know I couldn't. I am in awe that I wrote that last section. When we think our peace is about us, we feel the weight of doubt, but when we awaken to peace as a pure gift from God, we are free to receive.

It wasn't long ago that, when my pastor or my mentor spoke of keeping my focus on Jesus, I would humph more than a bit, and want to talk about my story, my transformation, my pain… and yoga. But that just kept falling away. Somehow, He must have always been with me before I ever became aware of it.

Jesus is the person this book is about because, at the end of the day, only God can help us discover the feel and the sound of what is most genuine within (heaven), in a newly opened realm.

Jesus is the person who is the logic of what it means to be human. Getting closer to Him will reveal the ways you may be far from your true Self. Why do you think we so easily forget the bible told us we were made in the image of our Creator? I have a number of Jewish friends who may prefer to replace the names Jesus and Christ in this book with 'the One' or any number of Old Testament names like Yah Weh. I'm confident no offense is taken (by God).

The next logical step is to vow to let your life love you. Yes, let your life love you. As your West welcomes East as a new mindset, you'll discover the wonder and beauty of establishing a covenant between yourself and your life, rooted in one underlying reality—*love*. For there is no 'I' writing this book that wants you to believe like me. There is an

I AM flowing through this human vessel inviting you to experience and taste the truth of unity with God, with life.

It just so happens that a state of love and protection is already present in the heart. Together, we can uncover it. I am here to share my story of hope and healing for anyone cycling through patterns that appear unbreakable.

Today is fresh and different because of Christ's in-breaking of love

nothing is the same

how could it be?

you are in a new moment

that was a breath

you've never taken before

can you see + feel your way to an entrance

a Peaceable Kingdom

where there

are no

locks

or

keys

Customized Compassion

Some of the phrases and words I've chosen to use in this book might get you feeling that you needed to have read the bible, read it more, or wish you'd paid attention in Sunday school. Nothing could be further from the truth. Simplicity is key.

There might be times when you picture me waving my arms in a charismatic action. Well, that wouldn't be unrealistic, for those are shapes too—and I love cheering on the world.

Please keep an open mind and don't be too concerned with the names I use to refer to that which is sacred. Language is a celebration, completely made up by hu-mans. Huuuuuu-mans. The first sound, 'huuuuuuu' is said to be sacred. Try saying 'huuuuuu' aloud a few times.

I am committed to blending a version of reader-friendliness with some scripture, as I invite you to understand the Eastern mindset and embrace Eastern practices. View it as a challenge and opportunity to yield the left to the right (here is your first brain reference, left brain to right brain). Shift from comfort or complacency to revelation, to more .

Just as the sun rises in the east, East will now be the metaphor we use to mean your growing awareness of being loved by God, led by His Spirit. Through this, you will see that your mind of Christ asks your physical, emotional, and intellectual selves to submit.

Rituals allow us to drop into cycles and seasons so that we can see patterns.

Now, about those waving arms—mine... and those finger-circles I asked you to make around the words yes and no. Those movements have a rhythm and are holy in that they contain the energy of life.

Even the turning of these pages or the 'click' that turns them for you is sacred energy.

And, guess what? All of this—the sighing, the circling words, the Huuuuuu-ing—all of it is your yoga. For what point is there to movement if not to be mindful of its purpose? A walk, dancing, swimming, golf... the list is endless, I know. And in all of this, in all you do, are you present? Are you joyful? Feeling your body's power? Are you in relationship with your feet, noticing your repetitive patterns, allowing the flow to bring you to a state of deep Zen-like inner quiet? Or are you like I was for so long—burning calories, fighting imaginary battles in my head, wishing my life a different one, wishing I was different.

Welcome to the church of you. It's never been about one hour a week in a pew, or thirty minutes a day on a mat—those are part of it, but it's truly about your relationship with the world during your waking hours.

How we do anything is how we do everything. Everything is sacred. You are sacred. You are holier than you think.

Remember the popular message from A. A. Milne's Winnie the Pooh: "...promise me you'll always remember: you're braver than you believe, and stronger than you seem, and smarter than you think..."

Does it excite you that you are holier than you believe, more sacred than you seem, and more conscious than you think? Make some more circles if you like. Draw a massive heart over this paragraph. Whatever you feel.

What excites me is how much you will discover about your true Self if every day, for one month, you bring your whole Self to your day. Five minutes here and five minutes there, living fully in the present where there's no distortion from a traumatic past interfering with reality. How's that sound? You- clear. Less clogged.

I'll invite you to participate in some strange ways—like potty breaths— you, present and breathing into your belly while on the toilet. Or you, regulating your nervous system in tiny increments with humming, instead of scrolling on your phone. You, taking the steps to trust your inner knowing, for the time has come for Jesus-followers to move beyond head knowledge. Now is the time to drop into your heart, into your gut, and experience the Life of Christ ever more profoundly. The truth desires to dispel all our fear. The Word, trapped between the pages of a book, liberated Himself and is delivering peace as a person. He does what he wants—He is the living God. No one can stop the power of a love which steps through the walls of your heart.

Many things you do on autopilot will become intentional—more enjoyable, allowing you to be fully awake and childlike. *Woke*, like my own sensitive and present young adult children call it. Many things we think come from conditioning, not from our own imaginations and creative centers.

You're going to read the word 'self' in this book many times. Sometimes it will appear with a small 's' and other times with a capital 'S'. Can you take notice of when your ego wants to think this self is in charge? Can you trust that we are referring to a self who is, was, and always will be rooted in Christ's love?

Kamikaze Yogi is an invitation to an embodied, East meets West path to awakening. Ultimately, as West, you will get to know East through what is unfamiliar, provocative, and often weird.

For so long, I wondered where I could find God Monday through Saturday. Now, during a global pandemic, no one attends church on Sundays. This has become a problem for those who want church on Sunday, for those to whom church is only on Sunday. People are demanding to return to gathering for worship instead of acting like the church and creating a new expression of love. The time is ripe. I was in search of the 'how to' of experiential faith and am honored to share that path with you.

The other day, I was putting together food packages at a local food bank. I'd wanted to volunteer during the Covid crisis, and here I was. I thought about factory assembly people, and how they might be doing repetitive movement every day. I wondered what meaning they gave to it. Over a series of hours, I watched my arms move and my wrists bend, and my fingers sort, and suddenly I was aware of my putting hope into boxes, and my repetitive movement was every bit the dance.

If we would apply this concept to all tasks, we'd see the light from our heart as our hands assemble products, type data, sweep floors, or cut hair. No action is insignificant. You, fueled by purpose and intention, aware this fuel's substance is love, is a desirable connection to the Self—give it a try, for this connection is of Spirit, the realm beyond the physical.

Putting on the kettle, making a peanut butter and jelly sandwich for the kids—every one of your actions is the dance of life. And when you know that, then you are fully present.

So why aren't we enjoying being fully present? Why don't we know we can retreat to silence and stillness to be filled? One reason is because we have so many unmet needs and unprocessed memories. So many darned thoughts getting in the way of the moment, distorting what is 'right here'. We were told Jesus was up ahead preparing a place for us in heaven. He himself tells us there is no future moment where you will be happier or more connected than right now. His consciousness is always coming down to meet us right where we are.

You and I are gamechangers. That is true. We are also shapemakers. And the awareness of shape making is life changing. Your life is worthy of change. But you must desire it.

Say 'yes' with a big check mark, right here

Passion In All Its Glory

Christianity is in love with Jesus, which is love-ly, but oftentimes disconnected with the body for fear of the 'flesh'. The word 'flesh' in scripture was never meant to refer to the physical body, but used to describe the ego when it is separate from God. This is an important distinction as you move forward with this book in exploring your physical body. For me, yoga led to the end of body chastisement.

Remember: flesh does not equal body.

As a good Jew, Jesus was probably bowing, kneeling, raising his head to the sky, even shaking/quaking, as the latter is an ancient Hebrew faith practice.

Today I watched a YouTube video created by a Black dance troupe of tappers performing an expression of lament in response to the murder of George Floyd. While including speaking the names of the others who've died in recent years from police brutality, this group, comprising ages 1—61, made it clear that the body is to be included in our healing. The body, which safely holds our ancestors' pain along with our own, must be permitted to be seen, and be part of our prayers.

How does that make you feel—placing yourself out there to be seen by others, by the I AM? Write a word right here about your feelings:

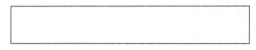

A lot of this book is about how we use our energy, because so much of the world is bent on destruction through words and actions. There is energy locked inside each body—we can grow toxic within if we don't learn to flow and feel some of the emotions like grief, impatience, unworthiness, and victimization.

We are redeemable. Always redeemable. *This book is 'rooted' in redemption.* My transformation and ongoing growth, my welcoming East into my West, has opened me to make what might seem to you, dear reader, wildly controversial.

The bible invites us to 'be in the world, but not of it'. When I embraced that, I began pestering Jesus with a question: How do I do this? I continued with questions including: Jesus, can you show me how to live without sin?

For a long time, I didn't know that to be human is to sin, and that it's okay to sin. I didn't know the power was in the repentance, the turning toward Him.

Startlingly, sin's shame became lost on me. This is a powerful concept I'll cover later in this book—one that I could say is about power, because when we talk about energy, we need to remember that energy is power.

Your anger = fiery power, your grief = liquid, cleansing power.

Power equates with choosing. I want you to see how amazing it is to become an energy converter. My desire, as you discover your emotional energy, is that you trust you can convert it (or drop it) into glorious action, divine inspiration, and sacred intercession.

Having reached this spot in my r-evolution, I ask no one say: 'goodie for you, Anita'. Instead, I encourage embracing the good and goodness for yourself. Imagine the end of criticizing yourself? In Christ, our domination mindset over our innocent body screeches to a halt. Black and brown bodies oppressed by systems created to crush might find it challenging to enter what's been stored.

As a survivor of sexual abuse, I know well the pain of this path. I also know that the journey from pain to peace does not have to be heavy, it is meant to be empowering. It's a love revolution in nurturing the Spirit!

I just finished reading *Going Home by Jesus and Buddha* by Thich Nat Han. He spoke of how people come to Plum village looking for peace and healing and to try on Buddhism. But ultimately, they know they need to go back to their roots, for that is where they find themselves.

The route to our roots knows many paths. Those people who went to Plum village can find how they belong to themselves. We are no different. We simply have to be willing to journey. Jung said that basically our Western psyche can't put on the full Eastern hat.

What we can do is embrace the East. And when we do, we evolve to a new breed of hu-man. Renewed.

May you journey to the other side of the Jordan, or just around the corner, to where that which you might see as ordinary love, intersects with divine. There's a perfect spot at a sidewalk café from which you can take it all in. If you like, bring along a towel or a mat, and your open mind and heart. Oh, and don't forget the tissues.

My wish for you, dear reader, is to fully experience this hu-man journey.

By the way: East will never ask you to abandon West, and neither will I.

In the Fire of Truth

Not that long ago, a photo of me with my family represented every bit the poster people for the good life. As a stay-at-home mom, my life had every creature comfort. But my inner life didn't match the image. I moved about with undiagnosed complex post-traumatic stress disorder (C-PTSD) and ADHD, resulting in an overactive ego for protection. It manifested in my body as infertility, tooth loss, chronic physical pain, mood swings and lots of other psychosomatic illnesses. I was a big personality with loads of opinions, low self-awareness, and I often came across as self-absorbed.

If I were to regale you with the abandonments and abuses I've experienced, and invite you to be a voyeur in my life, you might decide I have every reason to be a fearful, hardened and bitter woman—and that it would make sense to stay stuck in my sad story. Fortunately, my story changed, and I now celebrate triumph—good over evil.

The dis-ease we experience is often indicative of the choices we make and the emotions we process—and how we process them. My journey, like those of many people, required and still requires an adventure in uncovering truth. That uncovering of truth can seem a terrifying ordeal—and is so often incomplete. If only those venturing down that path knew who walks beside them, who dwells within them, they would never harbor fear nor doubt.

I got high once in my late 40's—seriously, I barely inhaled. Can you see me smiling at my own little joke? Anyhow, that plant medicine had a message for me despite me despising it's lethargic impact on my normally vibrant spirit. I sat stodgy on the couch while my friend danced around the living room, but what happened next is magical. I was shown an interior vision of energy coming in through my heart. This block of energy traveled down to my lower body and 'warmed' me, then made its way to my head.

You bring in pain through your heart too. If you do not have the capacity in the moment to process fully (not many do), then that energy gets stored. I was shown that my body was learning how to digest what came in, and to trust, without excessive armoring and fear. Thinking and thought alone cannot change without movement-releasing the deep emotional stress we carry requires effort.

Some common ways the body speaks to us include:

- An anxious feeling in the belly

- Migraines

- A phantom UTI (as in, feels like a bladder infection, but is not)

- A heavy womb

- Chest pain, stuck feeling

- Difficulty breathing

- Achy joints

- Inability to find our words

What pain are you bringing along every day? What pain is hidden behind the picture-perfect moments?

If you can bring yourself to share the answer/s to the above, in a word or a doodle, be brave and do it. Admitting can be the first step to freedom.

If you can't, can you circle some of the basics below? Make some shapes with your finger, a pen, or your eyes:

SOMEWHAT   SAD   MOSTLY   SAD   ALWAYS SAD

BACK   STOMACH   HEAD   HANDS   HEART

STABBING   SHARP   ACHING   DULL   STRONG

GRIEVING   UNSATISFIED   CONFUSED

ANGRY   SORROWFUL

Naming your pain or location, in the interest of changing your pain, is the beginning of its defeat.

The death of what you know is the best news and the worst news—a paradox—because ego will attempt to build a wall to avoid the shift, much preferring the status quo, but know that no walls will last in the soul—the soul will stand firm in the fire of truth.

We all have a natural source of healing energy/intelligence. I've learned: in relationship to God, so much of what I've needed outside of myself can be found within, with Him. I can connect to my highest Self and offer comfort and presence to the me in need.

In the East, it is known that each body has a series of energy centers we call chakras. Knowledge of these areas is second nature in the East. Chakras are focal points in the subtle body that were identified by mystics. Modern interpreters relate them to centers of electromagnetic energy—like a mini brain. In Western medicine, our body has a scientifically observed system called the endocrine system. There have been many scientists and doctors, like Candace Pert, PhD, author of *Your Body is your Subconscious Mind,* who compare the chakra and endocrine system. There may be more than 7, but I will focus on those main locations in this book.

"You just devote yourself to Me and I will free you from all sinful reactions."

BHAGAVAD GITA 18.66

The Gita is the yoga bible which is believed to have been penned around 400 BCE. In this verse, I found the underlying promise of daily devotion to tie in perfectly with my thought that people of many religions, of various ages, long to be free as promised by our one God, as stated in the Nicene creed, "We believe in one God, the Father almighty." Neem Karoli Baba famously said, "The best form to worship God, is every form."

Bring a soft smile to your face, now, while you form prayer hands, close your eyes, and allow awareness to drop into your heart.

What do you hear? Is He speaking to you from within you? Can you hear anything? A little? Not much? Depending on your own belief system you might wonder what in the world I am stating.

We can try another angle. Here's an invitation to the 'mind body yoking': stand up and shake. Yes, shake and bounce. Shake your hands hard like you are drying them in the air. Buzz your lips and stick your tongue out. Squeeze your shoulders up and down, then sigh loudly. Now, try going back to the awareness invitation to listen to your heart.

Write exactly what you hear:

Let's get to the heart of the matter. In the science and Spirit of ourselves, the heart itself emits powerful electrical impulses. It is the center of our being. Though every cell has incredible intelligence, the heart is the center of our physical and spiritual life, an organ of ethereal perception.

Remember when you were little, and told that Santa was watching your every move?

Yeah, my God is nothing like that… lol.

It's More Than Unrolling a Mat or Pulling up a Pew

If I had a dollar for every time someone has said to me: "I can't do yoga, I'm not flexible."

… I always say, "Well, that's not what yoga is about."

Sometimes they stick around and ask, "What is it about then?"

Well, it is about something pretty evolved. The amazing thing about yoga is that the practice meets you right where you are.

Many think that yoga is 'just' stretching. Health professionals, including chiropractors and osteopaths—many non-yoga teach-ers—tout the benefits of releasing tension in the body. My husband and two young adult children all practice some yoga. My guess is, throughout your life you've accumulated tension in your body—and stretching could probably help some of that tension. So, to some, yoga will not be much more than stretching. And that is okay. Yet yoga is so much more.

Over the past 16 years, I've been present in about a thousand public yoga classes, with dozens of different teachers, all over the country and, while some are purely physical, some purely spiritual, most are a combination.

Those who have touched my life are Christian teachers, Hindu teach-ers, agnostic teachers, and some who don't state their faith, and each gave me a piece of their heart. Add to that the overwhelming blessings

I have received in finding resonance with a number of Christian mystics. Through all that, I can confidently state the value of yoga.

The concepts here are likely new to you, but their power of peaceful practice can be easily absorbed with minimal impact on your time and maximum benefit to your overall, holistic wellness; an approach which supplements Western medicine and mindset.

In some way, welcoming East to your West is a guide—not unlike one you'd find from a travel agency that specializes in intensive explorations of hidden gems in known places.

You wouldn't go on a journey without some idea of a destination. Likewise, when you decide where to go, if its uncharted territory or it is commonly known to be misunderstood, you will probably talk to someone who has been there before, or who at least has some knowledge of the place. If the place is said to be a bit scary, it'd be nice to go with a friend. Going it alone, without any background knowledge, could be construed as unsafe.

Delving into your subconscious and energy body through the landscape of your physical body is best done with care—by linking yourself to someone with experience, someone who has traveled the path before you, someone who has experienced profound changes and is well- steeped in understanding the terrain. In essence, being introduced by a seasoned traveler (me) to the ultimate guide (Holy Spirit).

As your facilitator, I hope to reacquaint you with the guide who came before us, connect you to the person of Jesus who is alive and resurrected. He's going to welcome you to 'you unfinished'—and please, know this: the 'you (who is) unfinished' is complete. Confused yet? It's all good.

This journey: yours and mine, is collaborative.

Likewise, on our spiritual journey, where we invite East to join our West, we first find we must take small bites to digest the information. We also develop a new appetite as we awaken our spiritual taste buds. Let's agree to utilize this sense body to shape a renewed mind.

During our spiritual journey we will regularly find ourselves at cross-roads. We'll stand there and consider what we used to believe, whether we still believe it, and what we are willing to embrace. When we go through these stages, emotions we have not processed will surface. May you dare to wonder, "What if I am wrong?" May you wonder it often.

We, as a Western population, have a lot of undigested emotions. Why were they undigested? Because we have been trained to stuff down our right to feel deeply and to respond honestly. We have been trained to not have appropriate boundaries displaying inner authority. At this critical moment in history, the global pandemic and Black Lives Matter demand we explore our emotional bodies. This is likely new for most of us. It is likely the first time many of us have done this.

The more undigested experiences one has, the less energy one has to create, and to thrive. So many suffer fatigue, depletion of joy, or loss of passion, a sense of purposelessness. I have seen it many times; I'm sure you have too. It's easy to see that kind of thing in others.

It's difficult to see our own patterns, our own behavior. We identify triggers that cause repercussions that render us shadows of our true selves.

People who annoy us have the potential to be our teachers. But do we actively remember that?

Our laments are often stuffed down. They have been stored away for safekeeping until a time when we are strong enough to express them. But how do we gain the resolve to do that? And how scary is it to basically say, 'I'm growing, so bring on (and up) that which I've buried .' Just reading that might seem overwhelming.

But, once addressed, what was toxic in the energy-body becomes normalized: bitterness, hatred, and/or the inability to feel compassion or empathy. Of course, it takes energy to liberate ourselves, to believe that what Jesus promised is for 'me'... for 'you'. It's all energy work. It's okay, there's time. No one's holding a stopwatch.

So, speaking of that energy work, yoga is all about taking what we learn on the mat: deep breathing, balancing, stretching muscles to release their pent up 'old yeast', and using it to enjoy the present moment—all present moments—with renewed and deeper presence. Spiritual Self aside—even though it's never aside—the techniques in yoga help us break bad habits, eliminate negativity, and diminish stress. Looking back, it seems as if an entire decade of practice was used to heal my broken brain. Funny, I didn't even know—at the time—that it was sick.

Of course all those negatives would be reduced, because yoga is a spiritual practice based on harmonizing the mind and the body. It is an art and a science—isn't all life? It is a path toward healthy living.

The word 'yoga'—Sanskrit in origin—means to join or unite: on earth as it is in heaven. Maybe you have heard the term 'flow state', or even experienced it? It's a feeling of self-consciousness falling away, while being immersed in the joy of an activity or simply a state of being still. During flow state, time often feels like it has slowed down, senses are heightened, people feel at one with the task at hand and possess an awareness of fluidity between mind and body. Some people describe this feeling as being 'in the zone'. When we combine discipline with surrender, we give birth to flow.

During my yoga teacher training, I felt the call toward a merger of East and West. I stuck out like a sore thumb; the one who wanted to teach yoga in churches. Looking back, I think many former Christians were running as far from the church as possible.

I had to laser focus on what God wanted from Anita. When I did, he showed up on my mat, introduced himself, and referred to me as Grace. I took that as a middle name, realizing that this is what I was doing and intended to continue to do: extend grace. Actually, the name Anita means Grace. I hope I received a double portion. May we all receive a double portion.

In a master's level course on holistic Christianity, surrounded by women who were becoming chaplains, life sent me an embodied, Jesus yogi—an ordinary woman who was attending the classes. In a brief encounter during one semester, she changed the course of my life by suggesting I read a book: *Jesus in the Lotus* by Russil Paul. That book rocked my world.

After that, I gave myself loads of permission to be more playful and less fearful. Another big takeaway was that it quickly became obvious that I would not be called to live an inter-religious life combining Hinduism and Christianity the way Paul did, although I found it inspiring. During the time following reading the book, many people called this season I went through a deconstruction. To be honest, there was a period when my husband wondered if I was still a Christ-follower.

Fast forward one year.

I was teaching yoga in a prison for women. My heart had been moved for our growing mass incarceration problem. I met myself behind those walls in the faces of the inmates week after week. I met my own suffering Self who was 'herself-myself' hidden behind a thick wall of shame and pain. Then I decided to set her free.

One of the attendees said, "You know sometimes at night you are lying there and realize your own vitality as a sort of buzzing inside?"

She left it open for others to add uh-huh, or huh?

I was astounded. I was unaware that I had an internal buzzing but, upon reflection, I thought it must be kind of like feeling the engine of your own heartbeat, or like seeking your pulse then registering its movement and its spacing as one continuous hum. She had inspired me to seek something I knew would be valuable.

Yogis call this layer of energy within the physical—the subtle body. I have come to identify this vibration as the continuation of the 'big bang' in humans. Scripture says that, in the beginning was the Word (the Hum), and that Word was in God and the Word was God.

This energy of the Universe from 13.7 billion years ago can be felt in our bodies—how amazing is that? All energy is sourced in the one life originating at the Big Bang.

Mmmmmmm hmmmmm ammmmm ommmmm bzzzzzz

No words can capture

The Word... the resonance that's been

The river of the quantum field of interconnection since the dawn of time

Alpha

Creative energy

Sexual energy

Mental energy

Physical energy

Spiritual energy

Nature energy

Yet We experience them as separate and distinct

That is good

They may be of different vibrational speeds

And sounds

Expressed as unique

Dissonant

Frightening as in a lightning strike

And yet the safer and more whole

We feel in our nervous system

The more open we are to

Live as a *Yes*

For energy cannot be created nor

Destroyed

We are transforming

Harnessing

Purifying

Well, He is

I experience renewed energy through energetic practice. You can learn from this book, and much of what I have in this book is what I've learned from others. Others will learn from you. We become a chain of life-affirming information.

Go forth and seek by truly embracing this book—wrestle with the text, write all over it, read different parts at different times. Adventure, and challenge yourself to reach its peaks. Explore, and use what you find to drill down to your core. Create your own concepts using your own experiences. Drink it in as your elixir to life; an East meets your West cocktail.

KAMIKAZE: THE DIVINE WIND

There are many driven by passion—a desire for freedom—not just for themselves, but for the masses. Before I started the physical task of writing this book—the assembling, the collaborating with an editor, the going over scripture, the further review and extended study of East and West in many forms, and the physical practice and further education in yoga—I asked God a gazillion times why I was to write this book.

The answer came in various messages but, essentially: millions of rational people, millions of struggling people, have had a hard time uncovering the power and guidance of their own Spirit. And that is tragic.

The person of Jesus desires to be known in all, and knowing Him will restore the Spirit—that means yours, dear reader—through your heart. A restoration for the sole purpose of loving the world… and contemplate this: you are the world. A world, at one point, that was forged in the East.

Once I began the writing, I didn't need to ask any more. The world showed me that 'reason' in myriad ways. By way of the church I belonged to, some family members and folks I knew in my community came forward and, through their fear and doubt, and without knowing, drove me to question my role. Me, an ordinary woman named Anita, who received her middle name, Grace, while simply standing in mountain pose on her yoga mat, tasked to stay the course, do the work, feel the pain from her past and, most importantly, trust the messenger.

ANITA GRACE BROWN 43

This me, becoming Anita Grace, did her work, so she could do His work and, in doing so, realized those labors of love were one and the same.

But we struggle to accept that we can be so esteemed. Our brain-training tells us we cannot be one with God. As much as we wish to behold the infinite, the many faceted faces of God, we recognize within our Sonship yearning that we can never fully conceive the realm. We can be in a state of acceptance of knowing we are one and the same—therefore worthy of that state—and acknowledge an understanding that we are in shallow waters of the deepest lake of divine love.

In my growth, studies, and journey, I never want to leave my proclamations as final—I always want to restore mystery. Knowing Jesus intimately always equates to awe, wonder, and humility, Not assurance.

The West, when steeped in agenda/dogma, takes the Spirit out of life. The East returns it. As reliable as the rising sun, when East meets West, we are whole. Mind body is one. We exist in duality which represents the concepts that we require, a framework of opposites, in order to appreciate, know and/or recognize one or the other: good and bad, sweet and sour, deep and shallow, happy and sad. It is said that the awareness of these contrasts creates change. Think friction. Think iron sharpening iron. Think energy released.

Kamikaze means divine wind… and it means Kyle, which I'll explain in a little bit.

Divine wind? Surprised? Most think about the pilots who are often depicted in attack, in essence demonstrating strength, courage, and loyalty when they face a challenge to gain freedom—and pay an ultimate price. You, as an explorer of new attitudes and altitudes, contemplating adjusting your belief systems and journeying to new concepts, will require extreme bravery. Because step one was to proclaim: I believe in God. Now, our evolution is to explore our desire to experience what can never be fully grasped—a big 'K', Knowing, a first-hand intimacy with the I AM.

I have died a hundred deaths, thus far, regarding who I previously thought myself to be. These deaths are my leaving go of who I am *not*. I thought I was shallow, too emotional, prideful, lazy, not smart enough, too old, and yet, miraculously, the Father came and filled me with boldness, connecting my future with His ancient story. He does that every moment because I, like you, am worthy.

Put that helmet of salvation on your head, and be assured the Lion of Judah is all the protection you need to pass through dying to old versions of the self. I hear Jesus assuring you—there's no turning back now.

When I am bold, I acknowledge who I am—nothing left out. I am the bastard, the forgotten and abandoned, the broken, the sinner, the sick, the neglected, the addict (to my own unhealthy thinking). That is part of my messy reality which built the woman I am today. The treasure is in our innate ability to screw up, and do the work that makes us strong. In admitting I've had all of these labels, issues, and aspects—juggled them all, been almost crushed by them—it allows me to be vulnerable which, in turn, comes full circle and returns me to God. To not hide anything from God is to not hide anything from the Self. Choosing to love myself in all those places, I leave myself better than I found me.

As kamikaze yogis—yogis being those who practice yoga—we can put on our own armor in the form of the truth, truth as essential you, then come to understand that nothing can harm us. Yoga is one way for this corruptible body to put on the incorruptible Spirit. When yoked, the Homo Luminous, or torch bearer, steps forth.

"I think yoga is one path toward a consuming bond with God."

BEN WHITE, MY PASTOR AT CIRCLE OF HOPE CHURCH

If only there were more congregations that had leaders like him. And he keeps me in line. I paraphrase him: *you don't have to punch people with your message, Anita. Gentle goes the way, now.* He encourages me not to necessarily soften my message, but to ease the speed at which the concepts are delivered, and the language, all in the interest of people comprehending what I mean.

I may not always come across as ordinary Anita, and so I have people like Ben the pastor, and Marie the editor, to help me deliver the news. "Bring your reader to the kitchen table," says the editor, "the way you have been able to bring me there. Tell it to me, yes me, like I'm six," she has said on more than one occasion. "Put some of the pieces into stand-alone pages or read alouds, then be patient with how they are received," she says. "And, in the introduction, especially in the introduction, break all the rules and make it longer than most, so that people know what they're getting into." I have attempted to lay a broad, expansive foundation.

Just when I think she and Ben have been speaking—they have never met and are in different countries—she adds: "And, if you are going to bare your soul in an absolutely honest way that talks about sexuality, then show your dog-walking-self, cookie-baking-self too. And I mean it, Anita. For the love of God. Truly, for the Love of God. Because you know what, Anita? All this work we're doing together, and I'm 'getting' this stuff. I'm long estranged from scripture, and yet, with this East meets West, I'm getting this. If I am, then others will too."

And to that I say, "Amen."

And so, I'll be aware of my propensity to forget that I'm steeped in this study, and I'll remember that I sometimes assume people understand instantly, yoga or scripture. I promise to do that, for you, beautiful ones who are on the cusp of rebirth. You won't have to abandon Christianity to embrace the East. You won't be struck down if you practice yoga. I promise you that, too.

Kamikaze Kyle

"Death and life are permeable states because
the 'Risen Christ' represents to us everyone who has ever died."

I COR 15 (VERSION UNKNOWN)

Life is a mystery. Death, also.

Of one thing I am certain, Heaven would never be selfish and keep our loved ones locked away from us. Jesus' Paschal mystery (the passion, death, and resurrection of Christ—the work that God the Father sent His Son to accomplish on earth) is about much more than the miracle of a physical body resuscitated beyond the grave. For every human, there is a path of 'dying to the Self'. In Christian theology it is called kenosis (a Greek word meaning the act of emptying), and relates to our fears, and to the identification with a limited, disconnected ego. The word kenosis is used in Philippians 2:7, and says that

Jesus made himself nothing. The verse translates to becoming entirely receptive to God's divine will.

I imagine, on resurrection day, Jesus burst through each realm—from earth to hell, to heaven, and back to earth—to reveal to us what is possible.

My husband, Bob, and I have a GodSon, Kyle. Kyle passed in March 2019 after a courageous seven-year battle with a brain tumor.

Kyle, like all of us, is a child of God. God's son. In those final months as he endured suffering, those two words, usually with different meanings, began to merge, becoming one and the same in my breaking heart: Godson and God's son became GodSon.

When his body died, we experienced deep grief. In a time when we needed support from others, it seemed difficult for others to understand the effect of Kyle's passing on us—we were close. This was not the passing of an extended friend. There was a stinging pain to this; even our church family didn't seem to comprehend the relationship. It was painstaking to repeatedly explain that our grief was intense and prolonged because of this special assignment—that we needed prayers and care too. Over time, I have been able to show our community what it means to Bob and me to have a spiritual son. Once we see ourselves being God's child, we extend this to others much more readily.

Kyle loved to express himself with tattoos and, about a month before he left his body, I was visiting and he wanted to tell me about his next tattoo (his tenth, I believe.) On that visit, Kyle found it difficult to speak and became increasingly frustrated. Mark, Kyle's dad, told Kyle not to worry, and he pulled out his phone and brought up a picture of a skull with goggles and a helmet. It was a morbid image. For a moment, I was lost for words. Then I noticed the skull had a yellow scarf and so I said how much I loved the sunny color he'd chosen. But in my head, I was thinking: Kyle, *WTF?*

The next day, as I prayed for him, it hit me. That was no ordinary skull, that was a kamikaze pilot. I googled the image. Sure enough, plain as day, there he was. I'd missed it because I had been taken aback with the death imagery. I texted him excitedly: Kyle, you couldn't have known this, but that is the name of my book. You are getting a kamikaze pilot tattoo.

(Note: even before I knew what this book was about, God had given me the unique name for it.)

Kyle couldn't use his hands that well, he was limited to texting with emojis. He shot back a thumbs up. I typed back: We have such a special connection, you and I… I later wished I'd added: a soul connection…

And then he sent me a red heart.

Moments ago, I stopped typing this draft and went to my phone with the thought that the old text thread would be there so I could quote verbatim. But I found an empty thread. I burst into tears. Gone. Whyyyy? I wailed.

The day after the red heart text, I prayed for Kyle, again, and texted him: Buddy, you know you are not this body with an expiration date, a brain riddled with tumors. You are not a mouth that can't form words or hands that can no longer type. You are a soul filled with love, a Spirit which soars with God throughout eternity. I know he sent me lots of red hearts that day. My heart burst; we understood one another at a level beyond language.

Kyle's soul knew he'd put on his goggles and helmet to protect him as he traveled through the realms. No need to make that stop in hell since Jesus took care of that for all of us. Kyle was fiercely declaring: death has no hold on me. Death is not the end. What appears dead is only dormant.

Search for love beyond your fear and your limited mind. Enter your heart to discover a realm of heaven. Go searching, come looking, like Mary Magdalene did at Jesus's tomb. Look for evidence of Heaven in your life. Discover Him in your inner world.

Wherever there is beauty, there am I. Laughter, that's me. The break of dawn, me. A peaceful time chilling with friends, I'm right here. Tears? I am with you in your pain.

Know that this is Him, this is you, and this Him is in you.

These hearts of ours, these walkie talkie hearts that work as spiritual receptors, can receive the love of heaven and get you to feel it, all from the realm that Kyle now occupies. Heaven is within us. Heaven is now. It's a newly opened space from where grief dug its grave in us.

We may have had a fixed idea about our physical reality. We may be stuck in our Western brain. But we can change. We can and must lift ourselves out of our despair and continue our searching in the East.

Bob and I do it for Kyle. Who are you doing it for? Who will you do it for?

Out in nature, we'll find our nervous systems regulating, and we'll relax and get present. We'll invite the Spirit in and tell Her to have Her way with us. Enchant me! We consent to your action. We want to know about God's son. We shout into the void of the night sky: "What have you done with him?"

This speaks to Christianity rooted in wisdom and mystery, recognizing us as incomplete until love opens the door to connection to the Holy Spirit. Our Eastern practices bridge the way to what was always intended but somehow derailed. I recall many occasions where the Spirit required obedience; the 'go' to receive or serve in ways that I didn't often understand at the time.

Stand Alone

In the 1500s, Teresa of Ávila took the way of contemplation. Choosing the monastic life after a good many years living a reasonably comfortable life, she openly dipped into studying the mystics—and thus became one—and had no problem of meeting East with her West.

She said,

"The Lord is pleased to manifest to the soul at that moment the glory that is in Heaven, in a sublime manner than is possible through any vision or spiritual consolation. It is impossible to say more than that, as far as one can understand, the soul (I mean the Spirit of this soul) is made one with God, Who, being likewise a Spirit, has been pleased to reveal the love that He has for us by showing to certain persons the extent of that love, so that we may praise His greatness. For He has been pleased to unite Himself with His creature in such a way that they have become like two who cannot be separated from one another: even so He will not separate Himself from her."

You might think ego gets in the way of our journey to peace and divine light—ego is a barrier, even called 'the saboteur', to spiritual bliss, but Alan Watts, the writer and speaker known for interpreting and popularizing Buddhism for a Western Audience, famously said: "We are airy nothings".

It's true. When ego is in the way, it causes us to fear and control life. At those times, we feel small; we definitely get stuck in our heads. That's why we need an introduction to our body's ancient, reliable wisdom—which is why I'm placing you, through these pages, across from yourself to meet your hidden East Self. Some call that East Self your subconscious mind.

Have you noticed, no matter how much you 'try', you just can't seem to shift beyond certain bad habits, fears, or behaviors? It is only through the reptilian brain that a renewal of the mind—aka change—can occur.

The body cannot lie. The truth shall set us free. But first it will challenge our resolve and our determination to finish the task.

Trying to shift, thereby not shifting, but remaining in a continuous loop of try, creates a constant inner monologue of not being good enough. It looks like this: frowns in the mirror, absence from adventure, not applying for a certain job. It sounds equally pathetic when you tell yourself comparison stories: I don't have that quality so I'm a loser. I'm not gifted in that way so I'm not enough. You may have lots of stories about your body and its imperfections.

Can you see how that is not helpful? Are you willing to explore why it is not?

Your connection to the whole of your life is severely stunted when you do not listen to the truth of your body.

Shift requires action. Change goes against the body's natural system that wants to protect us from doing something differently. It's like the body says: 'Hey you're alive now, so why change? It's my job to keep you in a state of aliving.'

When you want to make a change, the body fails to see 'aliving' is surviving, and beyond that—with risk and work—there is thriving. The protection plasticity within the deep part of us doesn't go beyond that state of 'must protect from change right now' to compute that new actions stimulate growth to evolve.

After many months of writing and staying in the creative flow, I realized something had to coalesce to structure this book. When it comes to projects, I can be quite 'squirrel here, another one over there', which brilliantly feeds my creative Spirit, and is responsible for many wonderful projects and parties. It's on the sit down and structure that I can wane—especially in new endeavors. I prefer the active part of the creative process. Writing beyond feeding my creative Spirit would be, to have me 'not change'—the structuring requires me to make 'new shapes' with my life. Writing outside journaling would have me stay safe and not leap forward and ask, 'how exactly do I put my writing out there?'

By the age of 45, I had not yet found gifts and talents to share with the world. I was a devoted mother and wife, and I'd dabbled at many part-time jobs to supplement our income and stay sane. When poetry, then prose a few years later, began to pour forth, I was the most shocked of all. It must have been in me all along.

We all have repressed centers we can awaken. And guess what? When those centers are integrated, they are the purest thoughts, the purest emotions, the purest actions. I imagine that you, like me, have been searching for your soulful life; simply wanting to bring your piece of life's puzzle to the table and know it is more than enough.

New to 'put all that writing in a book', resolving to outline thoroughly, I went to my in-laws' home at the shore in New Jersey, and prayed the structure would form. Making that decision was a bit out of my comfort zone and a step in changing the routine and the way I had played (small) so far in the 'book creation' arena.

Suddenly, a chant came through me like a long-lost song. I replied to the air, aloud. Tears in my eyes and chills along my spine. I had tapped into my internal, powerful voice. I was on to something.

YahWeh. El Roi El Shaddai. Ey Yah Asher Eh Yah. Adonai. Jehovah Jireh. Shamah. Elohim (You can listen to me chant this on the book's YouTube channel).

These are seminal Old Testament (original) names for God. I was chanting names for God for some reason unbeknownst to me. Praise delivers a profound truth from within. Most, if not all, of the ancient names of deities are made up of sounds that have a vibrational essence which not only resonate within our bodies but connect us with all the vibrations that surround us. Sound made to praise God can create a bridge between worlds simply by our breath, our Ruach.

That reminds me, I was arrested a few years back with Rev. William Barber and the Poor People's Campaign. That day, I made fast friends with a self-proclaimed Jewish atheist man who promptly told me I had bright evidence of the Ruach in me. The Spirit of the Living One shines for people to see the holy Other is at work. It's more for them than us.

As an aside, Greek legend has it that, when a human came in contact with God, the human's hair stood on end. Of course, the hair standing on end is the autonomic nervous system's response, but how apropos that it was said to be linked with an encounter with the One. And how interesting that, when I prayed and the chant came to me, my nervous system responded to the sacred. Not just me, but many others' bodies responded in this way when I chanted this new (to me), ancient sequence.

And there we go: sacred not scared. The same letters, one position different.

I had challenged my inner self that wanted to protect me. I had made a change. I had stepped into a more linear but unfamiliar approach to my book project.

Talk about change. Evolution. If it can happen to me, ordinary Anita, it can happen to any human. Of that I am sure.

Understanding that my own tradition had names for God, powerfully grounded and rooted me in the Old Testament, preparing me to read the entire book in 2020. The names restore our connection to the Israelite within us—many still in bondage, pained from swimming in a sea of racism and broken systems. Chanting brought respite and, over time, restoration for me, as it has for many.

So I changed the way the book was going to be presented, so that it could reach more curious people. I had to learn to trust that someone would help me express my message—and I don't mean God.

Why is it so difficult to change? Because we are in bondage to our habitual behaviors and thinking. Our inner belief systems and coping mechanisms are conditioned -which looks like personality. For generations, toxic religion encoded a message of 'do not trust yourself'. I am here to remind you that no one gets to tell you how to process your pain. For no one has ownership over your body, your life, your sexuality, your faith. You are a sovereign being. You hold dominion over your own Self. Let that domination system from outside of you go.

Ask yourself: how much of what I think and believe is really me and how much did I inherit? How much of my life did I consciously create with desire and prayer and longing? On a scale of 1-10 how alive do I feel today? Most days, could I shout from a rooftop: 'It's the best day to be meeeeee!!'

Access your power.

Ditch the victim, the gossip, the busybody, the drama.

Turn yourself into your own hero.

There's a power inside us that is greater than most of us realize. We are conditioned to operate in low gear. Fear often keeps us from engaging a higher one. Fear and, dare I say, comfort. If we kick it up a notch, people will talk: label us heretics, question our sanity, maybe say we are getting too big for our britches. But it is our sanity that we are needing to save. Who knows, you might need to cycle through your 'John the Baptist' crazy for Christ season. Are you willing to do that for Him?

Teresa of Ávila was on the right track. She spoke of that superpower that can be accessed from within because 'it' is within. She said:

"Christ has no body now but yours. No hands, no feet on earth but yours. Yours are the eyes through which he looks compassion on this world. Yours are the feet with which he walks to do good. Yours are the hands through which he blesses all the world. Yours are the hands, yours are the feet, yours are the eyes, you are his body. Christ has no body now on earth but yours."

Place your prayer hands together and breathe—you are now yoking your body to your mind of Christ. It's that simple.

Struggling for Meaning

"For as long as the ego is the only self we know, we shall cling to her like a life raft."

CYNTHIA BOURGEAULT, EPISCOPAL PRIEST, WRITER.

Everyone struggles with not feeling strong enough to handle life. It's difficult always to be fully present. That's okay. I offer you the opportunity to practice tolerating discomfort by getting acquainted with it through anecdotes from my life; that way you'll feel safer in exploring the energy of an inner life that is spectacularly yours—practice being the curious witness to your discomfort. Get familiar with what makes you feel connected and what makes you feel absent/distant.‑

There will be unfamiliar words that reference scripture. Roll with them. Adapt to them little by little. They may seem odd. It's okay. Maybe you are familiar with bible quotes, but new to yogic terms? Same advice: go with the flow of the new information. Embrace the merger—or give it a chance (or a chant). Your body, mind, and soul will thank you.

One of the things I was most surprised about is that the bible is told from the perspective of the poor, the oppressed, the enslaved, the conquered, the occupied, and the defeated. This is the mystery of how the Word is enlivened in my body. It *only* speaks to those embattled parts of me! So when I read, I pay close attention to what brings goosebumps and/or tears.

History was not taught to us via a neutral curriculum. We learned about the revolutionary and civil wars from the voices of capitalism on the move to domination.

The subversive, brilliant, and enduring power of the Hebrew prophets is that they wrote from a bottom-up perspective. So do I. Each day I announce to God my bold willingness to get down and dirty.

Practices that are predominantly Eastern can allow us to reduce the stress we bring in from and hold out to the world everyday. Low level stress builds up as energy and causes a multitude of chronic pains (for me it is especially IBS).

The scholar-practitioner in meditation, Christopher Wallis, said: "The energy body is really nothing but the psyche as it interfaces with the physical body."

There are many 'systems' in the body: endocrine, digestive, circulatory... but, of the nervous system, we often hear sympathetic and parasympathetic. Much of what we are doing in this book is 'massaging' the nervous system into a new state of relaxed receptivity. Let's have a quick biology review of two 'easy to confuse' terms.

The sympathetic nervous system prepares the body for 'fight, flight, freeze' response during any perceived crisis or potential danger.

It doesn't know if those situations are real or conjured; it simply responds. It plays havoc with the immune system if it is constantly being called upon to run away or fight. You will learn how to climb that 'ladder' to a state of calm social engagement.

The parasympathetic nervous system is one that stops the body from overworking. It restores the body to a composed state. Anything we do to keep this system actively turned on is good for us: meditation, acupuncture, massage, high-quality sleep, music, art, laughter, and a connection to our higher power. Nature is especially powerful in helping us live in the present—time spent in nature automatically shifts our nervous system into a regulated state—and from this place we feel empowered to respond rather than react from habit. When we practice a peaceful directing of our thoughts, emotions, and behavior it's called self-regulation. This is an extremely healthy place to live in and from but, sadly, most adults are missing this in our Western culture.

To begin moving toward this state, consider this: play is the antidote to stress.

How are you playing?

Getting into a parasympathetic-dominant state means the body is able to self-heal. For those who are chronically ill, battling disease and addiction, the integration of these practices with conventional medicine is a true East meets West effort to holistically heal the whole. The wisest part of me gets the credit for my not taking mood-altering pharmaceuticals. I could not tolerate them and ultimately realized the world did not get to decide I needed to be more palatable. I was the way I was because my childhood experiences shaped my neurology.

Your own energy is medicine. You are an overcomer of suffering and disease. Say it loud and proud—*I am an overcomer and take responsibility for my life and health.*

Emotions, bodily sensations, thoughts, connections to what's ordinary, can develop into relationships with an inner child landscape where you are one with the Father through Jesus the Son.

The glory of inner life, of the soul's energy, is 'lit up' from within. It is completely possible to awaken to this new reality.

> *"At no point do the resurrection narratives in the four Gospels say,*
> *'Jesus has been raised, therefore we are all going to heaven.*
> *It says that Christ is coming here,*
> *to join together the heavens and the Earth in an act of new creation."*

NT WRIGHT, NEW TESTAMENT SCHOLAR, PAULINE
THEOLOGIAN, AND ANGLICAN BISHOP.

Picture This, Please

Let's engage the sacred imagination, shall we?

Let's say you're blind and you wander into a room, with strange smells assaulting you at once—because you're blind, your sense of smell is heightened. There's fecal matter, urine, and blood. Sound is amplified too. A woman is obviously in excruciating pain, and you know this because of the squealing, grunts, and howls like you've never heard before.

You're so confused and scared that you want to run—at least a large part of you wants to run. But another part of you, an instinctual, ancient, wise piece of you, invites you to explore further.

You feel your feet on the ground, you take some deep breaths. At the speed of the most powerful computer, you calm, and a message bubbles to the surface that you can trust she is not in danger. You don't even have time to question that, you just know that you're in a different mindset from when you entered the room and experienced the smells and the screams.

With that assertion, a moment of silence is pierced with an infant's cry. New life has entered a pregnant mother's birthing process.

Relief floods your whole body—every space inside you now completely reassured, you relax. In addition to celebrating a new life, you are celebrating that you didn't 'run away'. You trusted your inner voice that was aligned with wisdom, and did not follow your reptilian brain.

Your fear was unfounded. You're so relieved you didn't run, for you would have missed the miracle of new life.

Just as the blind person entered the scene and made a decision which brought joy, if you had entered my personal-life story, midway, and only witnessed my pain, my confusion, my struggle, and fear, you would have questioned whether to trust my story of faith in the one who is calling me to total reliance.

And, based on that, if you had entered my story, midway, and not known how I have evolved, you would not be able to trust the practices on the pages that follow. Ask yourself—do I really want the objective promises of Jesus to be lived out subjectively? Your yes will allow God to work in brand new ways—forget the former things; you'll be invited to follow the wild goose (Holy Spirit) into the wilderness so God can build fresh streams in what was wasteland. For scripture reference, this is an allusion to Isaiah 43:18.

I was lost, now I'm found. You can find yourself, too.

Repeatedly letting go of fear and moving through cycles of 'ego death' led to a less scattered and truer me. You can make the decision today to invite the miracle of life to be experienced through the lens of the body in addition to mind—a downward access to understand yourself at a deeper level.

There is a participatory God who has guided my steps. Good steps. This Christ, these signs that appear, the logic of my life, desire nothing more than to help create order out of chaos, we either evolve or repeat. Our ability to be alone with the Self lands us in a startling realization that this body, this breath, and this mind are of our Maker; truly sacred ground.

We have come to believe the disorder, confusion, lack of peace, worry, and fear in the world in which we live are normal. They are not. What if you are meant to enjoy a spacious mind where the pause brings song, inspiration, answers to prayers, maybe poetry, and will guide your next steps? Christ's work on the cross opened heaven's gates for anyone to walk through. 'Inspire' holds the root 'to breathe or blow into' from the Latin. God's going to fill you with His will, His plan to love the world. Breathe that in right now.

When we align with the truth of our identity, we commit to untangle what is in our life. How do we do that? By allowing a little East into our daily lives, curiosity over judgment, and a desire for more of God's promises.

There are angles and alignments for your subconscious mind, a.k.a. your physical body, which re-organize you at a cellular level. I know, that sounds so weird, but it's true. I experienced it. One day, the Knower assured me that after years of allowing breath to lead my body, Spirit would lead my life.

Emotional storms might rage within, but won't have the final word. We have a God who leads us beside still waters.

A peaceful realm within you can be resurrected from energy you already carry in bodily-held tension and pain.

Oh, and by the way, as you work through this, as you shout, 'no—explain it to me like I'm six,' but then later say, 'okay I can see how that language connects me with my own internal ancient sage', know that there's plenty of space to jot notes or expand these concepts. Paper copy of the book? Use a pen. Kindle? Grab some paper or use your phone's notepad or recording feature for your input. After all, you're being invited to participate in your own life. You're contemplating having East stay a while, contemplating a whole new mind.

You can learn by doing this worthbook.

Great Expectations

At the beginning, you likely wondered: what can I expect from this book? Now, many pages in, stories told, and concepts introduced, it is time to zero in on those initial expectations and let them go at the same time. Your expectation for growth means letting go of many expectations. Confusing? Challenging? I hope so.

I hope you are challenged, dear reader, in the best sense of the word. When you are, you can expect to discover a depth of peace that you'll hold onto like a bulldog does with his tug toy. Yes, it will become that valuable.

As you hold tightly, you can contemplate the solidity of the person of Jesus. He is not an impersonal, ethereal Spirit. He is a flesh and blood man operating in you. I know this is bizarre, but I promise you that your inner child will love your playful attempts to imagine this as a reality in an unseen realm.

No doubt you will get some shake-up too.

Changing your life, merging your West with East, is not an Ikea instruction sheet to assemble a set of shelves. While it is simple once you get it, it takes some prep work. Okay, maybe it is like those complicated directions where the English version of the shelf assembly instructions were not placed in the box of one-thousand parts.

I'll keep this short.

Yoga is not about the shape of your body, rather it's about the shape of your life.

Expect your parasympathetic system to be in full working order nearly all the time, and your sympathetic system—that machine of fight, flight, freeze—to reduce dramatically. That is cause for celebration.

Expect to be enchanted by your own experience of the Self, who lives safely in God. Who would say no to this offer? Over the past seven years, I've witnessed more than 300 students and friends arise from corpse pose, the final posture in a public class, awe-struck. Many more listening to my podcast have reported interaction with the Holy Spirit in a unique and comforting way.

When you read this book, I want you to say:

"I feel like I just went to church, to the therapist, and to the gym!"

Why I Am Doing This

Because the world provides us tools that don't last

For example, Alcohol is a 'spirit'

It can change the frequency we operate from, temporarily

Shopping is a 'spirit'

It can change the frequency we operate from, temporarily

Food is a 'spirit'

... you get the idea

You are an intelligent human being

But

We all have a lower, carnal nature which does not KNOW Spirit deeply

It does not speak to, hear, or see what is lasting and what is ephemeral

So we keep going for our 'hit'

And then we wonder what's going wrong

Nothing

Nothing is going wrong

We are getting that which we seek

There is nothing wrong with these worldly loves

Enjoy them

Fully

But do not think they will fill a gap

That is only meant to be satisfied by

breath, nature, singing, prayer, poetry, art, music

These are the Soul satisfiers my friends

Seek them and drink them up!

And your 'Knower' will

Lift you higher

And higher

Out of the realm of suffering

For several years, my prayer has been to be able to share a message through a book that will help change the direction of Western yoga. That shift would see the practice ease out of being a billion dollar, somewhat elite industry, returning reverence to its origins; to become a daily way of a life of wholeness: mind, body, breath—without the added weight of lengthy or complicated practices.

One tweak in and of the body or breath each week. You, your physical self, dancing with the spirit/soul in the unseen—truly learning to walk by faith, not sight.

Equally important is that my message can shift the intimate, relational experience of the solid person of Christ Jesus. We can each live the following question within the community, as well as when journeying alone: who is this Son of Man? Is his power as potent in me as he promised? What does His life, His boosting my immunity, look like, *feel* like?

Lots of books throughout the ages have pointed to a theology of the character or structure behind our shared reality, often called God.

As mentioned, Kamikaze Yogi is an invitation to an embodied, East meets West path to awakening. The gospel of your sense body.

THE SACREDNESS OF SEVEN

At a certain point in this book, the chakras will come into their own sections. Seven plays an important role: seven chakras—the energy centers, aligned with seven Old Testament names for God. Further, Mary Magdalene's seven very-ordinary human demons/sins are uncovered as our gems.

The Jesus I speak of when I reference my personal knowing of this Son of Man—who would walk through the self-constructed walls of my heart because nothing could keep us apart—carries a love so strong. He told me, 'even your demons, my dear, could not keep me away'. Yes, that powerful.

Jesus' plan is to point us away from our sin to humanity's many spiritual gifts.

LIST OF 7 CHAKRAS

Violet	Crown	Higher Consciousness, Connection to Divine
Indigo	Third Eye	Intuition, Perception, Imagination
Blue	Throat	Voice, Expression, Sound
Green	Heart	Love, Union, Grief
Yellow	Solar Plexus	Personal and Divine Will, Power
Orange	Sacral	Creative, Sexual, Emotional, Flow
Red	Root	Base, Foundational, Earth, Security, Survival

On the theme of seven:

The seven OT names for God which were given to me in my meditations (there are many more): YahWeh, El Roi El Shaddai, Ey Yah Asher Eh Yah, Adonai, Jehovah Jireh, Shamah, Elohim.

The seven demons/sins of Mary Magdalene: fear, greed/lust, shame, grief/envy, lies, illusion, attachment

As you journey through the chakra sections, may you feel confident that an eternal love is guiding you beyond your ego personality toward freedom—at liberty to be ever more the *you* were created to be. Begin where you encounter your own or the world's suffering and longing. A solid foundation of freedom supports your newly inspired endeavors.

Jesus is at work in our energy bodies (where matter and Spirit co-exist) through the Holy Spirit. Because of this, we are shown the kinks, the places where there is a block to the flow of living water.

We can use Mary Magdalene's healing as a universal, human template. As Christ is our blueprint, we can ask that our growing awareness reveal how we may need help in untwisting our plumbing.

As complicated beings who require more awareness, it is as if we are spiritually constipated by our inherited operating system, and suffer further complications because of our lifestyle and habits. We need the divine carpenter, I mean plumber...well, you get the gist.

Many ways of our modern life can make us feel we are far from our Abba (Abba is a word Jesus used for Father). I use the pronoun He and Father to align with the relationship Jesus described with the unseen, the heavenly consciousness. Many are bringing awareness and equanimity to God also being our Mother and choosing She. Mother is rooted in the word matter and so *she* is everything seen. We live in a Christ-soaked universe. All matter is infused with Spirit. Or, to put it differently, Mother is always fueled and filled by Father. They operate as One on earth and in heaven. Feel free to play with the words for God!

I have a respected friend, a body worker, who tells me with regard to the Trinity: Soul is Jesus, Body is Father, and Spirit is Mother. I like that a lot.

Many of us have thought—and many still think—our unworthiness is a strike against us, because we have to stop sinning before God will love us. But that is a flawed assumption. God demonstrated eternal love for all humanity when Christ died for us while we were still lost in our misidentification.

> *Jesus did not point to the sky when*
> *He gave the address of the kingdom of God,*
> *he said, "The Kingdom of God is within you"*

LUKE 17:21 MIRROR TRANSLATION, FRANCOIS DU TOIT

Taking it a step further, sin, misstep, error, is necessary for our growth. It seems that God is okay with that. We humans are the ones with the problem. It's demonstrated in scripture that he fully expects us not to be perfect, for simply to try is to grow. We are human, not God. God's love is within us and helps our being human. In the East it isn't so much good versus evil but ignorance and suffering versus wisdom and consciousness.

So if unconditional love is directed at us from God, why don't we feel it?

The path of a kamikaze yogi travels with the light into the deepest parts: our chronic pain, addictions, fears, manipulations, ignorance—right to the center of the suffering self, in the shadow. And that yogi travels not for navel-gazing, but to extend supernatural love toward the inner child and the Self who has forgotten the true nature of humanness. Maybe we don't feel that unconditional love because we are too far West.

Warming You Up

A review already? Well, we've covered a lot of ground. Consider this an expansion. Most often, yoga is referred to as a method of physical and mental disciplines. A man who practices yoga is a yogi and a female practitioner is a yogini. For ease, to include all, we say yogi. The word yoga comes from the Sanskrit word yuj. It also means to yoke or to bind. It is often interpreted as the union of opposites.

Masculine/Feminine

Heaven/Earth

Dark/Light

Black/White

Conservative/Progressive

Inner/Outer

Human/Divine

Energy/Matter

Young/Old

Rich/Poor

Future/Past

Doing/Being

Moving/Still

Personal/Universal

Deep/Shallow

Circle one word in some or all of the pairs that you most identify with. Now, look at its opposite. It may well be what you are out of balance with. Know that yoga will help you balance what you deem its opposite. The creation and expansion of the universe, through our growth, is derived in unification. Is that asking us to do yoga? Well, yes, I'm pretty sure it is. Yoga is more than a commercial marketplace of fitness routines. It is a sacred communication, a prayer practice to create a whole you.

There are western world variations of yoga which are class-roomed for profit, and made trendy for status. But, before any of this, there was simply a sacred, ancient practice which represented union, harmony, and peace. It was benevolently gifted and, at its core, its true meaning was not meant to be appropriated for commerce.

Here in the Philadelphia area, and other parts of the country, yoga is quite elitist with classes around $15-18. But I have always been called to bring the healing practice into the inner city and prisons as a volunteer or by donation. It's the same with this book, a way to make yoga accessible to all people.

Yoga allows us to make connections (the logic or logos of the Self) to our deeper layers, inner child, and potential future Self. As you develop this relationship, you will probably find that beginning to say

no to others, creating healthy boundaries, is the same as saying yes to
yourself.

It's amazing what yes to Self and no to others does. Decades of chronic
IBS drove me to find relief, and ultimately led me to discover healing, connection, and some magic. I found that through growing vitality, my own energy medicine and health, I could thank a Jesus who
was (and is) not shackled by doctrine. Yoga became a communication
channel—a two-way system—a mirror in my heart.

Sometimes though, when I'm ready to embrace the next brave thing,
I'll go back to feeling that tension arising in my belly, so I put my
hand there and I talk to myself. Then I breathe deeply, and relax my
face and shoulders. Sometimes, when I'm driving in the car, the tears
come, and I whisper to myself: I got you. I will never let you go.

When I do that, I'm talking to that hurting one inside, that brave one
who's not quite ready to grow up or be integrated. I am learning how
to smile to my own sorrow. We have unlimited little ones to reparent
within. Yoga helps us do that. It leads us to our first,true parents.

I saw and understood that the great power of the Trinity is our father,
and the deep wisdom of the Trinity is our mother, and the great love
of the Trinity is our lord; and we have all this by nature
and in creation of the substantial parts of
our souls.

JULIAN OF NORWICH, ANCIENT MYSTIC

This means we enjoy infinite opportunities to grow and transform.
SAY aloud: I am not stuck. I am not a tree. I, like Julian, am a hu-man

'unlettered', maybe even a wo(man) who is often known to be emotionally raw, yet has intense courage in my convictions.

When you engage that communication channel, your own heart like a walkie-talkie, you are not stuck.

With myself, when I talk to little Anita who is hurting, I tell her she can take all the time she needs.

You can try it too. Say to yourself:

> There's no rush
>
> you don't have to be a tough cookie
>
> you get to be a little one for as long as you want
>
> sigh…

Talking to the Trees

Within this book, you'll see the sign: Read aloud. When you do, it is the opportunity for the ultimate personal performance. And a bonus if you move your body at the same time.

I'll remind you, each time, that it's okay. It's only you. Stand, open your mouth, open your heart, participate.

Go read aloud in nature. Everything is alive.

Remember a song with these lyrics: I talk to the trees… but they don't listen to me…? Well that is what we've been led to believe, but it's not true. The whole world is listening with an energetic ear, feeling the vibrations. Be childlike and engage. You know who else talked to the trees? Mystic, author, philosopher and civil rights leader, Howard Thurman.

"If you want to find the secrets of the universe, think in terms of energy, frequency, and vibration."

NIKOLA TESLA, SERBIAN-AMERICAN INVENTOR,
ENGINEER, AND FUTURIST.

Read Aloud

It's okay. It's only you. Stand, open your mouth, open your heart, participate.

We're not meant to go through life zombie-like, helpless, without sufficient inner-resolve to reveal the hidden truth of our beloved nature.

Our Abba speaks this message through my heart...

I connect you to these women through your wounds
    to raise you up together.

Not on my watch.

Not to my daughters. No, what evil meant for harm,

I have reversed.

It is Finito!

You shall never see yourself as a victim again.

You are Victorious!

Up indicates movement.

It is my strength,

My power,

Which brought you up into the kingdom realm beside me.

Enjoy your nobility.

He's made us His own.

Each day this relationship shall deepen as in marriage.

To be brought up out of Egypt is to awaken to life,
    to God's power in you.

Your energy is love.

Follow the call all the way to full liberation.

You might want to go back to Egypt,

back to sleep,

where you were numb,

where you were a zombie.

But you are headed to the garden.

You'll commune with Jesus and the father—all day long.

You'll be cleansed of every wrongdoing.

You'll enjoy the truth of your own son-ship.

You can never go back to someone else's fairytale.

You'll live in your own gospel story.

You're the heroine.

You carry the promise of nobility.

Shame and fear can never hurt you again.

Once you've crossed the Jordan,

you are responsible for leading others through the mess,

until everyone is bearing their own fruit,

until you are the bride in the arms of your groom—

penetrated by his gaze.

Remembering To Thrive

Gehenna. A place in Jerusalem. In the Hebrew bible, it was where some kings of Judah sacrificed their children. After, it was said to be cursed. In rabbinic literature, it is said to be a destination of the wicked.

We have no idea what we are carrying, nor do we know what to grieve. Many versions of our old Self pile up like bodies in Gehenna, trapped, unreleased.

That frozen-in-timeness can be unearthed and dug up from under the weight of anxiety and fear. It must be brought into the light of day, this crucial sense and experience of one's own begotten-ness (properly Fathered, not an accident, not a bastard, nor a mistake). What is asleep inside is hidden from our view.

The layers grow, thicken, form tension, take on armor, and add weight, physical and emotional. This is why, when you look at the cross, its arresting image is meant to impact your psyche; you allow the anguish for the innocent one to draw forth. With dedication, patience, and compassion, our bodies will eventually reveal and transform the blocked energy. Keep looking into the face of Christ until you see your own twisted face.

The solution to healing and embodying the soul is not to engage the pain body (death of Christ in us) directly, and not to dig at it. Any attempt at confrontation only causes the pain energy to expand (maybe this is what Jesus meant in the parable of the demons multiplying? in Matthew 12:45). Instead, we can heal by focusing on actions in and of the light. Things like: the arts, nature, our pets, creating beauty, journaling, music. One study even found that time in nature for PTSD suffering veterans (formerly, only given pharmaceuticals) created an almost 30% decline in their symptoms.

These and other similar pursuits draw our inner attention to peace, not to struggle. In this way, the life-force gently squeezes out the memory of pain so it does not feel threatened or confronted. Our ego and our body each have many inherent protective defense mechanisms. Yoga comes in subtly with alternatives to our addictive behaviors. It replaces the good that became poison with the better. Our original needs were innocent, but our misdirected focus grew the weed instead of the good fruit.

Any version of the kingdom of heaven, any life of the Son in us, must include the entire path of Jesus. It must include the Good Friday suffering and death. It must include the Holy Saturday journey into hell and waiting. And yes, finally we get to experience resurrection. Suffering is our starting point. Suffering: during a global pandemic, witnessing continued violence against Black bodies, unemployment, medical diagnoses.

We first exhaust our attempts to cheer ourselves, then we suffer, and finally we emerge to a real and lasting hope.

I followed Him into every hell till there was no one left to battle... or blame

All of the devilish parts of me were integrated and belonged at home in my body. One day I woke, and the Knower assured me that I would no longer be needing to fight, that now I was free to dance with the divine. I thought- hmmmm, I feel married in my soul.

We have been lied to, and believed that our yes to follow Christ, to believe some creeds, would keep us safe from suffering, would protect us from dying, and would make us happy. The idea of the human Jesus now being in our own heart's heaven, in His resurrected state, comes as a shock to many people, including many Christians. Where else would we find Him?

I cannot tell you how many times I was saddened to hear my fellow Christians say, "Jesus is coming back for us." When I know He is back and I've had the pleasure of learning how to rearrange the furniture of my interior house so that He might find a comfortable space.

We are missing two-thirds of His journey. The kingdom of God includes all of life and, when we can get fierce with reality and begin showing up for what sucks, then we will find our way to Sunday. We wander and wonder why life feels so dissatisfying, ordinary, and repetitive. Where is the newness? Where is this evergreen life blossoming up from the soul's winter?

We will learn much as we begin to observe, then embrace, our own weakness, inflexibility, discomfort, imbalance, even our cellulite and aging. Love is there. A personal aspect of God has not abandoned us in our crazy-making.

We thought we were being protected from the world's pain with our armoring, looking the other way. But no, our bodies were open and interacting all along, a cell within the whole of humanity's body.

It is our lonely mind which could not tolerate the grief, the fear, the jealousy, or the lusts (simply our human demands—I must have this *now*).

These desires of the first three chakras are primal; what makes us truly a rare breed of human is our ability to *aspire*. These 'first three' point to what is ours to do. (We will discover each chakra, in depth, soon.)

Four hundred years of 'I think therefore I am' has led our rugged individualism into lonely silos of thinking we could keep gaining without ever having to lose or let go.

We thought, in stuffing it down or numbing with alcohol, food, and Netflix, that we'd avoid pain and live in survival mode. But we know exactly from what we are hiding—a sexless marriage, a burgeoning credit card bill, gambling. But there is only one way, and that is through the pain. We are stronger than we know. Let us remember, we are here to thrive. Are you with me? Together we will secrete our secrets and seek optimal health and wellness. This is God's promise: the balm of Gilead is Jesus, your medicine in the form of cleansing and anointing.

Read Aloud

It's okay. It's only you. Stand, open your mouth, open your heart, participate.

What did Yoga do in actuality?

Unfixed my identity. Put Jesus at my center

Destabilized the ways I saw myself which were not serving
   the highest good.

A purification of the heart.

I had come to love (and trust) God enough

That in the midst of my longing

I grabbed the caged bars over my heart and tore them apart

with my bare hands,

Revealing what was behind the desires driving my

destructive tendencies,

Exploring what those desires had been feasting on.

I had to break my own heart—

and surely it was God who asked me to self-destruct.

Jesus who threw the first stone.

On this journey of union with the unseen Father,

we will all be given the opportunity to sever in two

the personal will which had been

forged when we thought we were on our own,

forged from control,

forged from fear.

Sure, she's a human and she's being breathed by the earth,

but what of the moment of consent when she allows God's breath

to expand and contract her lungs?

Who is she then?

She is primal nature,

Dancing with Spirit,

Merging all supposed opposites, creating a whole woman.

She embodies her own Soul in this life,

Not content to wait to resurrect in an after-life.

Boom!

Dear reader, right after that last line, shout Boom and claim as many of the above words for yourself. Let's do it. This is a read aloud.

Breathe in. Get ready. 1, 2, 3:

I am not content to wait to resurrect in an after-life.

Boom!

SPACE FOR MAKING SHAPES

It's difficult to read instructions at the same time as making shapes with the body. For this reason, your phone can be your best friend. If it does not have a voice recording app, many are available as downloads. One such is 'easy voice recorder'. It's installed quickly, is free, and simple to use. You can also use your camera's video to record your audio. The great thing about recording the instructions for movement is that you can play them more than once. You can amass a whole collection of practices. I have also recorded them for you on the book's YouTube channel.

Making and keeping any small promise to ourselves is always a new beginning. It's a chance to carve a brand new neural pathway. Each time you get up and try is a cause for celebration. Here I am, cheering you on, arms raised over my head, shouting, "Yes! That's exactly it. Just keep at it."

Learning to LET GO/Flow

Stand and take a wide stance (this can be done seated as well).

Close your eyes and take a big breath in through your nose, then loudly exhale or sigh out of your mouth.
Do another two big breaths and sigh with each exhale.
Next, while breathing comfortably, swing your arms from side to side—first slowly, then after about ten swings, go faster.
Do this for about a minute or two

Now, come out of a swing of arms and, as you inhale, reach overhead, spread your fingers wide, and squeeze your shoulders up, feel tension.

Drop the shoulders and arms and exhale.

Flop! Slap those arms by the side

Repeat. maybe even 3 more times
Now, with bent knees, breathe and drop the head heavily.

Bending forward—as if there are hinges on your hips—fold over.

Remain folded and hanging forward for about half a minute…
inhale let, exhale go —in through the nose, out through the nose, now. In the warmup, we let some exhales out of the mouth, then generally we continue the practice all through the nostrils.

Slowly, bring yourself from bent forward to standing—in a bit of a roll up—ensuring your feet are grounded and steady.

Ask yourself in a moment of pause: "So, what's happening now? After each of these spaces for shape-making you'll want to let your body absorb what you experienced.

You do this by lying still in corpse pose for 3-10 minutes and grounding. Grounding is your connection to your body and the earth. Corpse posture is the most important of all. We agitate our energy during the practice, shaking and loosening then, ultimately, allow our nervous systems to settle. We move from sympathetic state to parasympathetic. We go from mindful movement to mindful stillness.

We are reconditioning what we might be used to. That 'what we are used to' is often rushing and distraction. We are practicing presence and allowing our brains to release all those yummy hormones like oxytocin, dopamine, and serotonin which naturally lift our moods.

Part 2 Shower Ritual

Create something like this when you are in the shower.

Please take away
All that is no longer needed
Within me and around me
So I may be left
With your presence of purity

SPACE FOR MAKING SENSE

Do you have a question? Is there something—a name, a concept—that you want to remember for later? Do you want just to stare at the page and allow yourself a space to rest? Have the urge to trace your hand? Go for it. Maybe you used to do that as a child.

Question: are you the person you thought you would grow up to be? Are you living the life you'd imagined? Why or why not?

This sacred space is for you. Fill it however you like. Draw, doodle, journal, list…

THE CHURCH

In the book of Revelation, John writes to the seven churches. There's that number again. The essence of revelation for this book's purpose is about the chakras, your spine being the reminder you are akin to being a whole book of God's energy. Just as chakras are energy centers, so are churches.

The energy centers in our body remind us we are full of life and of love. They may well be the 'seals' we read about in the book of Revelation. When we are firing on all cylinders, and our communication channels are open and flowing, then our life is revealed to be complete, because Christ completed us—He completes that circuit.

The East recognizes seven energy centers in humans. In moving away from its mystic roots, Western Christianity has forgotten or abandoned them. For those of us who want to mirror the church in 'themselves', to speak to a restoration so that what's out of balance can be restored, we can say the church within is real. It always has been, it's just that the meaning has been corrupted over the years in power struggles and battles of ego.

The other night, at the church I've attended for three years, a man who's been coming for eleven years announced, "I am the church, and I bring who I am to a space so I can activate love to operate it in that space, to help and to share, and we are all doing that."

What a concept: that we are each the church, that we each bring who we are to a space in order to activate love, to operate in love, through love, in the name of sharing love.

I thought that was tremendously insightful—worth repeating: we are each a church, and we bring ourselves to a space where we can activate love. We activate that love to help and to share. I am doing that in writing this book. You are doing it by reading this book.

God sanctifies or heals my chakras with yoga, and informs other people's journeys in other ways. I just keep doing me. You do you!

Since this man so cleverly introduced this simple yet deep concept of church, I've asked myself what I can bring to the world to activate love. Where do I take my church?

The obvious place, to me, is in the community and, if I remain authentic and open and serve others, feeding them with my gifts, then the embodiment of church is a success.

If you are a church, and your life—as the Karla Anderson song says—is a cathedral, then where do you activate love? Where do you take the church of you?

Where do you share the news that Jesus came to liberate you from the captivity of the many worldly domination systems?

Where do you work out your salvation with fear and trembling that it is not simply a personal matter of a heart change?

The local church body has informed this book. *Kamikaze Yogi* carries truth because I humbled myself to others. I didn't sit in the house and write for over two years; I wrestled and cried over what was ready to die, finding death before death found me. All so the new thing could be born.

I agonized—blood, sweat, and tears—so the world could read about my Jesus.

If I hadn't been called to that church, I wouldn't be writing this book.

"For Jesus is not another religion, Jesus is what God believes about you."
FRANCOIS DUTOIT, MIRROR BIBLE

Recently, I had a collective memory of all those months of me asking, "God, why me? This is too painful." God told me, on those occasions, that it was because I, like many others, was strong. Because he chose me. Because this was an honor. Because he believed me to be able to carry the truth.

And, guess what? So are you, dear reader.

We all have that power to help free the world. Anyone who thinks for themself and invites others to do so, is magnificently dangerous… just like Jesus. I find our problem is we just don't go far enough in our bold explorations. We get frightened of what others might say. Empires demand you follow particular orders.

It's a common question. Not always directed to God, but certainly up the perceived chain of command. How often have you been mired, or are mired, in the 'why me'? How much collective time have you lost to the 'I am a victim'?

How can you flip it?

What I learned about the 'why me', is that I would often attach it to the 'helping others and that which they needed to be saved from'. Of course, this was presumptuous. But, at the time, it felt good to be 'saving' others. Instead of guiding, or leading by example, I managed to get involved—entrenched, even. During a long season, I projected a savior mentality onto other people. My need to play God was real. I am so sorry.

So sorry.

What an error in judgment. On many levels.

What I truly needed was to back up, and remember that is not my role.

Eventually, I did.

I backed up to save my own inner child, so that when she grows up, she will be human and not God.

There is incredible freedom in stepping out of the role and back over the line to humble servant, worshipper of wonder, and stayer-in-my-own hu-manness. So much less pressure than trying to be God.

But of course, I'm playing Monday morning quarterback here. You can't see it when you're in it—thank goodness for coaches.

Our faith is filled with a built-in schizophrenia. Everywhere we turn it's 'don't play God', but in saying that, some leaders are doing just that. We also hear 'be Christlike'. And that gets confused with playing God. To be Christlike is to be self-emptying of our divisive nature, our former, unhelpful assumptions about how life works, a reality rooted in the world's greedy, busy, and distracted culture.

In essence, we need only to be human. Think of it this way. Be Christ-light.

When we leave the familiar, it takes a long while to find our people. The yogis laughed at the foolish Christian, for certainly they'd moved beyond that (and it hurt like hell). Then the Christians were mistrustful of the weirdo yogi. I had to keep moving beyond the world's rejection and suspicion, forging my own path from an inner resolve to trust Him.

Jesus is the light, the energy, and the power. We are not Jesus, we are each a witness and a lamp. We say to God, 'I consent to your action, your wisdom, your presence be done unto me. I am not the do-er. I make space to receive.' Oftentimes, He is an unidentifiable force, an 'other' life, a Zoe life, in us. If you've ever been pregnant, you might recall that bizarre reckoning with self-surrender to this new, growing life that you cannot see, but that you can feel. This is our faith in our own instincts, tears, and goosebumps relaying truth. The world of physicality will demand proof no one has. We, the artists, the empaths, the musicians, and the yogis are holding keys to an aspect of reality few are willing to explore for fear of being called crazy. I see you. I am you. But for so long, like Jesus's friend Lazarus, I was asleep.

I thought I was 'them'.

Communally: When God calls us to participate in the resurrection, that means we, like the witnesses of Lazarus' arising, are responsible for helping to remove what binds others to death. We must get messy and move closer to the stench of things like addiction, homelessness, and sex trafficking, in order to loosen the ties that bind in order that our Jesus' incarnate power can crush the principalities which have brought nothing but destruction and weeping.

For us, personally:

That we have more to learn, and can grow, is a good thing. It is an evo-lution. The world we live in is one in which we think everyone needs to be saved, but the real growth happens when we direct our energy to save our 'Self'. It is caring for the divine self, the soul which certainly for a season usually involves boundary setting, which to others may appear 'selfish'. It is what we have to do to be truly alive. Saving the Self is necessary growth, and so is being saved. That way, when we present ourselves as a church, of service to others, we come from our own fullness.

We work on the Self to be good for the world,
to become human, not God.

The evolution of spiritual virtues is always a gift to the world. For example, I asked some friends to join me in praying for President Trump. One woman reluctantly agreed, replying: 'Soon I was crying, struck by how difficult it was for me to pray for DT as God would want me to pray: to pray purely, to pray without asking for what I thought DT should do, or for what I thought he needed, but to pray in love.

I shared with others how humbling that exercise was for me, to purely pray for the 'enemy', how I wrestled with my own ego . When I told my friend Lorraine (a Black minister) about my struggle, she sug-gested that, perhaps because of privilege, I have not really had to pray for my enemies. She explained that praying for our enemies has always been part of Black spirituality. "We're used to that. We've always had to do it," she said. That was a profound revelation. This story moved me profoundly and I share it with you to encourage you to trust God to move in your heart when you show up and pray.

As we progress to become the most human we can be, that's when we're closest to sacrificial love. At that point, we're not working on a hidden agenda to play God.

The new breed of human has ears better able to hear love and suffering, and a voice stemming from a heart connection—an extraordinary phenomenon unfolding.

I have always found it curious how at the resurrection, Jesus said to Mary Magdalene: "Do not hold on to me."

The quest for sovereignty will demand we journey alone much of the time. It is not unlike a sacred sabbatical, or time in solitude, our own exodus from toxic relationships and herd mentality. All of this solitude assures you that your reliance on the One will become certain. All this solitude reveals there is only One voice left to trust.

Before the crucifixion, Jesus spent time alone in the desert in contemplation. After much prayer and fasting, He encountered Satan's temptations. You too will encounter your own 'demons'. You must decide whether you will trust Jesus that they are powerless; a venomless snake.

The path to enlightenment takes many forms, but it is almost always solitary—or contains great periods of alone-ness of thought, as well as physical distance. People will leave—it will hurt. However, you will see the logic when your emancipation is ever-present.

Take all your human idols off their pedestals. There is no need to play God. There are infinite reasons to be human.

SPACE FOR MAKING SHAPES

Balance

The cerebellum has 70% of the brain's neurons. Since I recently discovered I'm healing from ADHD, I wanted to share that physical challenges like balancing and coordination for 10 minutes twice a day, will stimulate the brain's parts which impact ADHD, especially.

Tree pose

Standing now press your feet down and find a spot (that's not moving) to gaze at.

Then, find your breath: in and out.

Now, picking up your right foot, place it back down and, using your imagination, say: I plant new, deeper roots in love and safety.

Take your left foot and make a kickstand with your heel against your right ankle, then reach your arms overhead forming branches.

You can keep your left toes on the ground or balance by placing your left foot against your right calf. If you want to put your hand on a wall, feel free, for this is your practice.

Stay in this pose for about a minute before repeating on the opposite side. Have fun. Ask yourself: What kind of tree would I be?

You can do different things with your arms too. Prayer hands. One arm up and one down.

Pray

In my heart yes, and in every cell of my being
A mind quiet with peace
As it's reminded of the divine
The truth of my own Being
Please reveal yourself to me
Sweet friend, my Jesus

Are you blind?

"Blind Pharisee! First clean the inside of the cup and dish, and then the outside also will be clean."

MATT 23:26

SPACE FOR MAKING SENSE

Do you have a question? Is there something—a name, a concept—that you want to remember for later? Do you want to just stare at the page and allow yourself a space to rest?

This sacred space is for you. Fill it however you like. Draw, doodle, journal, list...

THE CHAKRAS—THINK WHIRLPOOL

Chakra is an Eastern term that helped me understand how the energy is organized in my body, and how excesses or deficiencies have contributed to physical, emotional, and spiritual suffering and well-being.

The seven chakras are named, but are often referred to by their position.

The root chakra is the first chakra. Feet to cervix (in men it's feet to the anus). Its color is red and its element is earth. Postures that are associated with root chakra are those which ground us and bring about nervous system safety, anchoring in a solid sense of Self.

The second chakra is referred to as the sacral chakra. It comprises your sex organs. The color associated with it is orange. It is characterized as being of 'water'. Flowing movements are referenced with this chakra—non-linear movements. Dancing by accentuating a swirling of the hips, bouncing with a soft belly, and buzzing the lips will allow a sense of softness and openness to enter.

'Personal Will' is the third chakra. I call it divine will. Most refer to this chakra as the navel or the solar plexus. It encompasses the digestive system. Yellow in color, fire is its sign. Postures activating the power of this energy center announce: 'I will bravely step into the fire of awareness, simply to burn up what was never true.' We strengthen the core of Self with a focus on our strong center.

The fourth chakra is heart. Its location is obvious, given its name. Its color is green, as in 'ever' green. The sign associated with the heart is air. The heart chakra encompasses the lungs, and heart energy is rich with the sensation of a refreshing moment. We might find ourselves saying, 'I have never been right here, right now, and that newness brings me joy.'

The fifth chakra is the throat chakra. Represented by blue, it is associated with the element of ether. We give voice to our deepest, truest Self, expressing with words, song, and sound. I found chanting to be one of the most powerful practices to balance this center.

Sixth is the third eye chakra. It is between the eyebrows. Its color is indigo. The associated element is light. When we close our physical eyes, we activate the third eye and light of the heart which connects to glands in the brain—pineal and pituitary. From here, we see with an enhanced ability. In a paradoxical vision, two things can be true at once. All confusion drops like heavy rocks to the bottom of the ocean.

Moving to the top of the body, and beyond, is the crown chakra. It is exactly as it is described, 'at the crown of the head'. However, it doesn't end, and goes up and up and up into the cosmos. Crown is violet and associated with bright light and golden light—as in pure light.

As for the entire spectrum of chakras: imagine the rainbow of ROYGBIV from bottom to top.

On the colors: If you are like me, one of those people who do not see color when you close your eyes as related to the chakra, fear not. While each chakra is associated with a color, they are powerful enough without having to associate them with color.

Of the Chakras

The chakras are whirling pools of inner energy in our subtle body. Have you heard the saying, 'God's gonna trouble the water'? Well, right now, with the world upside-down in a pandemic, and a burgeoning Black Lives Matter movement, I do believe that God is externally allowing us to see incredible injustice that has lasted centuries. He is troubling the water.

Internally, our own bodies reveal imbalance, either an excess or deficiency due to life circumstances, trauma, or the conditions can be inherited, unhealed wounds.

We bravely enter our body, wondering why the chronically painful upper back, the migraines, the IBS are a part of us. Some ask, why are our lungs where we get sick first? Oftentimes, it is stuck energy, ready to be released as we process grief and unforgiveness.

Our chakras are said to vibrate at varying speeds, based on the rainbow, from slow red at the root up to the fastest violet at the crown. Some say, "vibe higher" which means don't be dragged down by negativity and worry. I like to think of the lower part of the body being the bass note and that we shouldn't have a preference for 'higher'—I believe that thought process is a recipe for spiritual bypassing.

Lowering into our guts, our sex, our roots are where we will discover the answers.

> *"For an angel went down at a certain time into the pool*
> *and troubled the water;*
> *whosoever then first after the troubling of the water*
> *stepped in was made whole of whatever disease he had."*

JUBILEE BIBLE, JOHN 5:4

Questions

One of my first yoga retreat teachers, Jennifer Pastiloff, author of *On Being Human: A Memoir*, asked us three important questions in a certain order to ponder our identity.

Here's the inquiry:

Answer in writing here—

Who does the world say you are?

Who do you say you are?

What is the truth about you?

Healing

We all have a natural source of healing within us.

"To lose our connection with the body is to be spiritually homeless."

ANODEA JUDITH, AUTHOR

The 'bible' on chakras that most yoga teachers recommend is *Eastern Body, Western Mind*, by Anodea Judith. It's not just for teachers; I highly suggest it to anyone who is interested in understanding inner child work, the nervous system, and ancestral body memory.

Other than for herself, your yoga teacher does not hold healing powers and cannot heal you. The healing powers do not belong to the rich tradition (of yoga) in the Hindu religion, and do not exist in the Buddhist philosophy which yoga often mimics. The healing power is held within you, and belongs to you. It comes directly from God.

You just don't understand energy.

These five words bubbled up from my Soul the day I followed the call to leave my yoga teaching jobs and trust the creation of this 'book baby'. I never swim. Ever. But that evening, Spirit called me to go to the nearby indoor pool to swim laps—crying all the while—and hearing this message:

We are pulling up shallow roots, my love.
Together we are laying deep roots. Writer's roots.

There I was, gliding through the water, when I heard that in my heart. I brought my head above the waterline and looked up. There I was,

under the banner of Lane 8 which turned on its side became the infinity sign. Warm tears trickled over my cool, chlorine-water-soaked face.
Awestruck. I experienced a depth of knowing that somehow, beyond
my wildest imagination, I'd be writing my first book at 52; and not
just any book; it would be about God, and it would be very, very bold.

I would have to learn to trust the process.

When you make shapes with your body, you will be engaging the
chakras and, through this reading, you will understand how that
engagement will help you. Remember the mention of letters to seven
churches? You'll be attending all of them within your body.

All mindful movement has been a wonderful way for me to hear soul
messages more clearly. You are likely to find that, too. When you
begin making shapes with your body for the first time, or make more
shapes with your body from a different mindset, you will become a
better listener within and without.

When I did this, I realized that qualities I deemed in myself as negative
my entire adult life, ways I told myself I was a terrible listener, were a
sign of undiagnosed ADHD. They included: oversharing, interrupt-
ing, dominating conversations, being distracted by background noise,
having a hard time remembering and inattention, having 'no filter',
talking too fast, rambling, getting off topic, forgetting what I was
about to say, being too unfocused so that I couldn't find the right
words.

Is this you? Or someone close to you?

What a miracle it is to trust our own innate intelligence to heal and become a discerner of the one true voice which resonates with eternal love.

When your Spirit pays attention, you will soar.

Claiming the Voice

I am the most ordinary of the ordinary. My story is a belief that if this unique voice of divine love wants to speak through me or anyone, He will speak through me or anyone. And He does. We just don't hear that voice because:

We just don't understand energy

The thing is, we don't know what we don't know. We cannot see, we are blind. Then one day we grow more curious and less judgmental. We make the decision to journey into our Selves, burrowing a path in the dark toward what we pray is a solid center. For the world is filled with movement. What the world needs is more conscious movement, more intention.

We begin to understand a little bit about energy

Once I embraced a slower pace—the pause of breathing deeply, and mindful movement—I realized I was responsible for getting to the root of my mood swings and my inability to be fully present.

I began to understand a little bit about energy

For those of us with complex PTSD—which comes complete with a manufactured mark of unworthiness—the messages can flow through us as magic. Our bodies, filled with chronic pain, cry out for relief, and cells attack themselves in a last-ditch effort to shout:

You *just don't understand energy*

And so, little by little, I began to understand energy. Physiologically, traumatized people have had to exit the building (the body) in order to survive. It's time to come home.

My nostrils flare as I write this, my body confirming truth. The Soul within each one of us is one with the Universal Soul. While many are seeking healing through psychedelics, the psyche—meaning: the Soul—can be embodied safely through these practices. Experiences of unitive consciousness change us at a cellular level—our minds never go back to being fragmented.

"Do you find reality harsh—so harsh that the mind has to be fragmented in order to fragment the pain?"

GABOR MATE, SPEAKER, AUTHOR, PHYSICIAN.

These moments of mindfulness allow us to draw forth the greatest potential in ourselves so that we can experience oneness with humanity. I underestimated my sentience and, in so doing, often operated from my lower nature. This is not a problem for God since He is the One in Genesis who clothed us in 'animal skins' in order to cover our shame. We simply must learn to shed this layer.

It is said that Jesus has always been coming as the doctor for the sick. We are invited to explore physical sensations, unhealthy habits, and conditioned thinking, where we might be hiding an unmet need.

And when we explore and release, suddenly there is an obvious disconnect between inner life and outer life. Upper life and lower life, life from the holistic right brain (where it is thought that trauma is stored), and life from the logical left brain. What is said is not in line with what is thought. What is thought is not in line with gut instinct; the instinct burrowed deep: in hiding. What is thought is certainly not in line with the heart's natural compassion. The compassion, nearly extinct, must be raised from the dead.

So much of what I intuit seems delivered from the mysterious place called the Soul. It often seems that expressing what is delivered makes me a freak. A Jesus weirdo. The shadows speak, the crows, the earth, the furry animals… all a language of love for me. I desire this intimacy for you; a love language flowing to you, a gift from all of nature seen through a lens of the new, old-earth.

I want for you a lifetime of mysterious and magical experiences like when I was out in my kayak on the river yesterday. I was loving nature—truly verbally expressing my joy to Her in the form of addressing the trees, water, sky, and hawk—when, suddenly, She mirrored love back to my heart. I began to weep. That feeling of being loved was a moment I won't soon forget.

ROOT CHAKRA—THINK MOTHER EARTH

When you hear or read the words root chakra, think 'ground', 'foundation', 'anchor'. The root chakra is referred to as the first chakra. Its name is exactly that—imagine a long line of your ancestors standing behind you, having risen up from the earth in the Spirit realm, cheering you on, shouting, "Be brave, we've got you."

Being disconnected from root chakra energy can manifest as high levels of fear or stress, addictions, depression, obsessive disorders, or an extreme need for control.

When out of balance, it's where fear resides.

Root chakra is linked to:

Survival

Security and safety

Basic needs like food, sleep, shelter, self-preservation

Physical identity and aspects of the Self

Grounding

Support and foundation for living life

So, with root being our survival and our basic needs, it's going to relate to our relationship with food, rest, and home; it's going to invite our return to the womb. A weak root will make one manipulative, insecure, pushy or operate like an 'unscrupulous politician'. I realized at some point that being a first generation American, a daughter of

German immigrants who arrived right after WWII, severely impacted the health of my roots.

In terms of ancestral connection: we are currently seeing a massive shift in awareness that African Americans may experience root chakra deficiency due to our country's history of slavery. There is so much healing to be done and we are ripe for it.

You will know your root chakra needs tending if you are generally sluggish.

To judge and disconnect from your physical body might sound like: I'm so fat, I hate my body. You might, even subconsciously, say to yourself that your body is a machine, its purpose utilitarian, an afterthought. Another realization for me was referring to myself as a 'tool' in God's hand. Again, this is about a relationship between persons. Take notice, is there a voice inside who dominates the body, bullying like a disappointed or mean boss?

The trauma and the abuses that affect the root include: birth trauma, abandonment, poor physical bonding with biological mother, malnourishment, early illnesses and surgery, any type of abuse, inherited trauma (survivors of slavery or holocaust).

Of course, energy overlaps or, more accurately, forms unions or relationships as the body runs as one physical, holistic system. But the underlying organs and foundational issues are separated by energetic chakra centers.

In Western medicine, we see doctors referring to the endocrine system to draw a location and symptom parallel to the chakras. Where the West seeks answers with and through medication, the Eastern approach is always: let's first try what is natural, obvious, long term, slow burning, not a quick fix.

Medical science recognizes those chakras—as your endocrine system: a network of glands. Each gland makes hormones that help with communication throughout the body, and aids the cells in talking to each other. They're involved in almost every function in the body. We are building immunity. How interesting that now, during Covid-19, we have increased understanding of how our immune system functions.

Of those cells: their state is either harmonious—healthy, or in protective mode—stressed. They can only be one or the other.

Stress disrupts the endocrine system's order which then can result in chemical imbalance—hormones produced, or not produced—hence, the communication system within the body begins to fail.

Anything we can do to destress those cells supports the whole body. So, what can be done? We can make shapes with our body—they've been doing that in the East for many thousands of years—that's right, yoga. Yoga embraces the power of the reset—creating coherence for the whole—and is a way of reversing the physical effects of stress, and the cellular response to stress.

Classical yoga includes a total of 8 limbs. This ancient system goes beyond making shapes, learning to breathe consciously, and meditating.

I would highly recommend you read more on the other limbs. Summarized: yama (abstinences), niyama (observances), asana (*yoga* postures), pranayama (breath control), pratyahara (withdrawal of the senses), dharana (concentration), dhyana (meditation) and samadhi (absorption).

Stressful energy comes from current stimuli, worries about the future, and is embedded, in a way, from past experiences. Our highly intelligent nervous system stores these experiences in the oldest part of our brain structure—in the limbic system which includes the amygdala.

All of this stressful energy compromises our performance, therefore our existence, by affecting our immune system. Stressed cells create chemical imbalance. In a state of imbalance the body does not communicate within itself from part to part, and creates chaos. When there's chaos, the door to disease opens.

Some things that compromise our immune system are: history of abuse, eating disorders, victimization, guilt, anger, regret, unforgiveness, unprocessed grief, and self-pity.

In dealing with the whole—and restoring balance—we work with the whole, yet can focus on the parts, starting with the root chakra. The characteristics of a person with a balanced root chakra are overall good health and vitality. Personal attributes include being comfortable in body confidence, a healthy sense of trust, the ability to relax.

You can have poor health and restore root connection.
Maybe you won't be traditionally 'cured', but you will announce
'I am healed because of a new relationship to and with my body.'

I learned a lot from the divine words which were messaged from God to my soul: My love lives in your pain.

Keeping in mind that the root chakra is located feet to cervix, (or anus in men), there is a big Aha! moment in that the heart cannot and will not blossom without a strong anchoring in security (AKA ventral vagal tone).

A few years ago, I happened to be reading an article and came across the word 'cervix'. I immediately felt nauseous, and began to cry. A memory from my childhood came to me. I suffered a number of traumas as a child. At this time, though, the memory was of something that happened when I was incredibly young: a caregiver had followed a protocol of administering an enema.

I saw it as an act of abuse I had suffered. I later learned that it was common in the fifties and sixties to give children enemas. In those days, it was not intended as anything but an appropriate way to keep children regular. It was addressed in the same manner as a 'take your cod liver oil pill' request. It was still a violation. It was not sexual abuse, but it was an interference with the body's natural way. Sadly, it was common. And it was of the times. I have since learned that many people cannot get by without taking laxatives. I often wonder what root chakra breaks they have suffered.

I had felt it as abuse, and my body, Spirit, and mind had regarded it as such.

Throughout my life, I had issues with my bowels. It is clear that these enemas created a root chakra break.

I relate this here because our memories, and the valid stories we attach to those memories, are the stressors that become a part of the disruption to the communication, to the healthy cells. So many early experiences impact us. It is an aspect of our taking on shame.

And they can impact us well into our later years. To this day I can't have a bowel movement without magnesium. My body does not know how to eliminate on its own. It's a chronic issue for me and, perhaps, for many others, too—many adults are addicted to laxatives.

Recently, I found myself in the endodontist's chair, tears streaming down my face in pain after five needle attempts to bring numbing—I was still experiencing a 'hot tooth'. In that physical pain, I was recalling the year before, overcome by grief in that very chair, as Kyle, our Godson, had just passed. My body remembered: I needed prayers, I needed relaxation. I scheduled myself a massage and lots of time reading and resting in our hammock. Teeth-Bones-Roots.

Root Chakra Story

I was in the basement, meditating in silence, when an online conversation from the day before popped into my mind—a conversation with one of our pastors on Facebook. We had been discussing the journey of inner peace and yoga. I'd defended myself and made my case. During meditation, when the conversation came to mind, I felt capable and empowered in that moment, yet there was something else that was like a loose end, something I was compelled to do, or feel, that I couldn't identify.

After the meditation, I got on my knees and decided to do 108 Ashtanga Namaskara, aka caterpillar, which is done by inhaling, lifting the seat from child's pose (into a table), exhaling while bending the elbows back, then surrendering the heart to the earth. Then, with strength, pushing the body upright and returning the 'seat to the heels' child's pose. The number is significant in yoga for many reasons, one being that the diameter of the Sun is 108 times the diameter of the Earth and the average distance of the Sun and the Moon to Earth is 108 times their respective diameters.

The decision involved effort, core strength, and determination. Somewhere along the way, I found, when I surrendered, I could dedicate each movement of strength to someone I love: a friend in need, a person in my small group... many others.

About halfway through, tears began to form. I had entered my heart. I could safely express what had been that loose end from the discussion: you are not bad in the defense of yourself, but you *do not* need to do that. God alone is building you and building your life, and so this is what repentance feels like, turning back to Him and His light.

Connection is a powerful thing. Connection to the Infinite in our finite Self. Those neurons fire back and forth—they are the logic of everything. Such was the case when I finished the entire 108 moves; I remembered the day that the call for the book came. I'd been swimming, crying, and hearing, "We are pulling up shallow roots, my love. Together we are laying deep roots. Writer's roots."

The message I received through this series, that I felt compelled to do after defending myself in a dialogue with a pastor, is that: when we defend ourselves, it is not good or bad. Some things just are. Non-judgement is the way to go. Once we purify the heart, we have restored our child-like innocence that Jesus often reminded us of in scripture. After this initial lesson, I found that I was given a few more opportunities in life to sit in my own natural desire to speak up in self-defense, but the Spirit asked me to hold tight within the impression of being guilty.

I understood, through this messaging, that the old was gone and it was time to create. All of us can be whomever we decided to be because, with God, all things are possible.

We are co-creators with God. Authentic roots are established by embodying our own soul. No one can 'see', with their natural eyes, your relationship with your body. Meaning, no one but you can know for certain whether you've connected in love or not. This relationship is healed in an instant and the shape or strength has nothing to do with this restoration. This yoking is an inside job.

You can purpose your life as you wish. The connections that were made during my physical discipline, when I dedicated them to others, was another form of communication—still from the same source of love—to serve others and send them prayer energy.

I commit to honor my ancestors and put down deeper roots for all. Roots that say 'Friend, you are good.'

Numbers, details, seasons, proportions, dates, and times matter to God. I was in a medical yoga seminar at Jefferson University with a renowned teacher a few years ago. During a seminar, he wrote '108' on the white board. When someone asked the significance, I immediately knew in my Spirit, but then that wasn't the answer the esteemed yogi gave. For my purposes the 1 represented how we start in life as separated—the me is a good building of a self. I believe my 'self' to be 'I' and I am in control of my life. Then the 0 is the kenotic space we enter when we submit to empty the Self, our pain, and the false ideas we took on for the sake of knowing God's truth.

Deconstruction has been a part of the Christian faith from the first words in the Hebrew bible where we see the letter 'shin' means to destroy as part of the statement 'In the beginning'. Instead of a constant renewal of faith, so many just kept building the ego as if the mystery were knowable. Becoming like a child restores our sense of enchantment with God. And what does the Word of God do over every destruction, every chaos? She, the ruach, the feminine wind/breath of God, hovers supremely with light.

Finally, the 8 is that God himself is rebuilding us into the new covenant, unity with the 'I AM'. Yoked to Christ, we are connected to the universal consciousness in our surrender to Jesus as King. We are whole. Infinity and beyond.

Stand Alone

God is so intimately knowable because one aspect of eternal truth is a person named Jesus. I have been asking, as I write this manuscript—who am I? Why did He make me a certain way: a woman in hot pursuit of agape Love? I have come to learn, to train, to partner. Educate me Lord. I am your echo, your mirror.

When I say that God told me, it sometimes surprises me that this statement is not more ordinary among my Christian friends, and I've been asking Him to show me why that is.

Throughout my 40's, He began my deconstruction—tearing down false beliefs, trauma-infused memories in my body, as well as all ideas of separation. Almost daily, I am filled with a deep loneliness that defies my reality. I am forced to my knees pleading with Jesus to invade the pain with his tender love, because I must carry generations of women's distraught belief that they are managing life alone... the adage that there are no reliable men left. A dark night that lasted a few years.

For maybe a decade, my les petite morts, mostly on my yoga mat, were energetic releases of the pain body—dying before we die as many have said. Truly the shrieking of a triumphant warrior demanding to be known as the Savior over the evil which had taken root. This sinful one who only had the capacity to serve self is gone. But the key here is not to judge this one who came before, this one who was doing her best, she who was comprised of raw material which became kindling. During that season, I often dreamed of carrying a baby both in my belly as well as in my arms—the subconscious preparation of my rebirths.

When friends tell me that I am unique, my reply is that I am not, that God is unique. Into my wounding He flies to make His home. The wound may be the entrance for the light per the poet Rumi, but it is also the entryway for the 'evil'. A woman in need of her carpenter, making all things new. Jesus asks me to help him build an altar on the place where He and I meet.

One comes to know, in a bodily sense, the prayer of Paul to the Ephesians 3:14: Out of God's infinite glory, may you be given the power through the Holy Spirit for your hidden Self to grow strong.

This hidden Self is being constructed bit by bit by our wondrous carpenter, replacing what I've surrendered. At first, before integration, the new inspiration is *all* God and then after much patience and prayer it becomes more me. But that has been a many year process even to begin to say yes to the empowerment Jesus has for Anita. Just last week I had the fascinating realization that I seemed to have returned full circle to the very person I started as- both wholly different and exactly the same.

Daily embodied practices which combine discipline, strength, balance, and surrender reveal the flowing, living water at my center. In solitude, the wild, soulful nature is welcomed.

Once we are 'found', we stop looking outside and discover His power is consummate, His fullness delivers courage, resilience, faith and, best of all, the presence of unshakeable, personal Love. You'll not only incarnate the body of Christ, but the Spirit of Christ and the mind of Christ.

You will know the excruciating leap from being saved to being Freed. Your whole Self is now set only on what Spirit desires, emanating from the unseen and eternal realms. If we continue to live in the shallows, unable to explore our own wounding, we will be left despising the wounded.

What the world reads as only hieroglyphics, our knowable God, through Jesus the Logic of humanity, reveals in a language only your heart can decipher. As you practice inner listening, you'll be receptive to more of this love language. But the noise will have to be minimized until you hear the pounding of your heart as the faithful servant hammering away a steady beat, a rhythmic reminder—I am alive in you.

SPACE FOR MAKING SHAPES

Imaginative prayer

Part 1: Take a seated forward fold. This looks like legs outstretched and your upper body relaxed and draped over, with arms dangling, chin dropped, and knees unlocked. Say aloud: the red blood of Jesus' sacrifice covers my whole body. I am cleansed and made new.

I am bowing to this reality and will arise humble and made ready to enjoy the strength of Him as Lion. I want to hear His roar in my jungle. Try sticking out your tongue and 'hahhhh'—a lion's breath.

Stay for as long as you like, repeating this statement and breathing calmly and deeply.

Part 2: Here's a little practice to be playful with your inner child. You can engage like you are welcoming an orphan or your own Self. You can even pretend you are talking to Jesus himself.

Prepare a warm, nourishing, and healthy meal. Something simple and delicious. Now, take the utensil up to your lips and say to this child, let's see now is it too hot? Shall we blow on it? Let me touch it to your mouth and see. No, it is just right. What do you think? Is it salty or sweet, creamy, or dry, chewy, or soft…what of the food's texture? Can you chew it slowly, enjoying the flavor? Do you love it? I made it special for you, honey. I am so happy you are enjoying it. I hope you can feel all the love I poured into preparing you something so nurturing to your body and your soul. Did you see the colors? I liked knowing I was making you a rainbow to make you feel special.

No

Find a quiet place and sit in a comfortable position. Do the best you can to relax your muscles.

Choose a word or phrase that has special meaning to you and makes you feel peaceful.

Or you can inhale… yah… exhale weh

Close your eyes.

As you breathe in, slowly produce the sound, Yah, as if you are sinking into a hot bath.

As you exhale, slowly produce the sound, Weh, which should feel like a sigh.

Breathe slowly and naturally. Inhale through your nose and pause for a few seconds. Exhale through your mouth, again pausing for a few seconds.

Don't worry about how well you are doing and don't feel bad if thoughts or feelings intrude. Simply say to yourself, "Oh well," and return to your repetition. No need to control thoughts but thoughts should not control you.

Continue to be aware of your breathing while you sit quietly.

Then become aware of where you are, slowly open your eyes, and get up gradually.

I recall many times in public yoga classes when the teacher would say things like the psoas muscle (located in the lower lumbar region

of the spine; extends through the pelvis to the femur) and the pineal
gland are direct connections to the soul. I am reminded of seeing
people with intellectual disabilities as being without ego and their
souls clearly shining forth.

Oh, how I longed to know my own soul!

SPACE FOR MAKING SENSE

Your sacred space for your questions, observations, and theories.

Writing Between the Chakras

Here's some space for writing, as provided before.

Here's the space to write those questions. This is the spot to freefall write all the things you didn't know your hands wanted to write. It's a breathing place. The rest between chapters. A place for you to create a prayer. Another sacred space for you.

In addition, I invite you to draw a representation of you, as you are now... a doodle, a stick person, a symbol of a portrait of you.

SACRAL CHAKRA—THINK PLEASURE

I prepared for this section with a little Van Morrison for dancing, followed by some tender touch to greet and thank my body—coming into relationship with her through sense-uality... not sexuality... although that would be fine too.

A balanced second chakra restores our right to feel. The gem of this sacral is creativity. Most hu-mans fear the energy in this chakra or they are being manipulated by its destructive powers. Many are addicted to porn. The world has seen sex slavery and rampant sexual abuses of every kind, even on children. I pray that sexual energy is harnessed and purified, and that those who are affected by depravity are able to experience a restoration of purity and creativity. My prayers are directed through my heart and via my writing.

The color related to sacral chakra is orange. Water is the element associated with it. The sacral chakra is all about flow and flexibility—in terms of the pleasure center, think about it being the river of you, a cleansing stream.

This chakra is located about three inches below the navel. In the back, it's right where your lumbar vertebrae are. Location-wise, some describe it as extending to the genital area, and at the level of the ovaries for women and the testicles for men. Imagine the pelvic bowl.

Sacral chakra is linked with the lymphatic system—the lymphatic system is a part of the immune system, an extensive network of vessels that pass through almost all of our tissues to allow for the movement of a fluid called lymph. Lymph circulates through the body in a similar way to blood. Lymphatic obstruction is a blockage of the lymph vessels that drain fluid from tissues throughout the body and allow immune cells to travel where they are needed.

It covers: emotions, relationship to the Self and other, expression of sensual pleasure, sensing the outer and inner worlds, and fantasies. We are repairing our disconnect from our five senses—what we taste, smell, touch, hear, and see—and brings us to a state of enjoyment through our body in an innocent and pure way. These practices of heightening awareness can help us to recognize unhealthy patterns in treating and/or ignoring the body.

Jesus helps us to end cycles of violence. For example, you might think of the guy who kicks his dog, the woman who can't stop screaming at her children, as external ways we extend violence in our frustration and stress because we cannot seem to process our hidden grief and rage. More often, however, I have seen it is more subtle. Our bodies take the brunt in a multitude of ways as the innocent 'me', (also known as my body), who must be punished.

When we realize this 'me' is in Christ, it is as if Jesus is speaking to us when saying: "You know not what manner of Spirit you are of". We are demonizing again. That realization grieves us and God. But I know we can live unburdened. We can live avowing: there is no one to punish, least of all you, oh precious and wise body.

This chakra's demons are lust and guilt. Early on in my writing, Spirit kept bringing in the words impotent and virile as they pertain to Jesus' power. If we do not let Him be Lord then we will continue to be burdened by lust and guilt. In the places where lust and guilt once dwelled these practices have now created a prayer life in me that is the life of Christ's Spirit. A movement of tears, words, laments, gestures, and other demonstrative moves appear and are permitted to be prayed through me. It is an honor to allow the Spirit to proclaim the mighty power of Jesus. It is an honor to wail and howl for the extent of injustice in our world—Lord hear our prayers.

We can state, "oh, being human means I've struggled with lust and guilt but now I am free." I met a man at a Universal Christ conference in NM with one of my favorite teachers, Fr. Richard Rohr. This stranger happened to tell me, in our five minutes together, that yoga was the practice which shifted his 'dirty mind' when seeing young women in their tight yoga pants to seeing them as beautiful and without lust. He said it was miraculous at his age of about 70.

When your sacral chakra is blocked or under-active, you may be experiencing a sense of lack of control, ranging from uncertainty to an inability to cope with life's changes. A person will become detached from their own emotions and those around them. A block is like a dammed stream of water.

Throughout my 40's I complained of not being creative. Suddenly, when this chakra's energy released, I entered a season of juicy and endless inspiration for my work. We do not exclude all of the energy of the first three elements of ground, water, and fire. They are the basis for the opening of the heart center.

Jesus wants our freedom—in our Spirit and in our matter.
He is the One *who floods us with HimSelf-Resurrection!*

With the sacral chakra, the first thing that comes to mind is a person's relationship with sexuality and how connected to pleasure and self-pleasure a person is.

"The flesh is the hinge or pivot of salvation." Tertullian's famous statement in his treatise on the Resurrection of the Dead is a powerful one. What if all our lusts have been pointing us in the direction of wholeness of soul the entire time? What if every time we feel the heat of passion arising, it is a calling to integrate a lost piece of our own soul/psyche?

We are built for pleasure. Connection to this center brings healing. Who wouldn't want to reconnect to this fountain of youth? It's regenerative and anti-aging. Our creator is forever young.

Gifts abound. Once, my friend called me a hypocrite. Her daring to speak truth in love turned out to be an incredible gift. Her insight allowed me to grow for: *"Faithful are the wounds of a friend; but the kisses of an enemy are deceitful."* Proverbs 27:6

So why did my friend call me a hypocrite? To put it bluntly, I was living a double life.

My friend was right. She was also wrong. Being a Christ lover does not mean perfection. It means we sometimes forget our real nature and find ourselves in need of God's love and mercy.

The other day I was biking and was nearly hit by a car as a young woman on autopilot went through a red light doing about 45 mph (in a 25 zone). She made a mistake. It could have been costly.

That moment made me think about the time when my marriage ran on autopilot (low awareness): I nearly ran it into a ditch.

God does not leave us where he found us. No, he has much better plans for his children than that.

With the chakra's element being water, the e-motion (energy in motion) is one of flow. Feelings are supposed to be flowing and unimpeded.

Are you connected to your emotional Self? Are your emotions flowing through you or do you feel stagnant, or even that a barrier is stopping you from flowing?

Sexuality and money go hand in hand. Keep this in mind when considering the aspects of this chakra. If you can't seem to save money, or you spend it frivolously, may the balancing in this chakra restore your self control because you are enjoying more conscious sex.

I was diagnosed with premenstrual dysmorphic disorder over 15 years ago: a complex condition. We now know the true diagnosis as complex post-traumatic stress disorder (C-PTSD) caused by many unhealed big and little traumas. The mood swings I experienced were severe, and some friends mocked me as being bi-polar because no one liked the fact that you never knew which Anita you were getting that day. Yes, my emotions were flowing, but they were out of my control. Once I addressed my sacral chakra and found healing, everything began to feel appropriately balanced. Anger flows, grief as well. There is no longer a wild rapids or an out of control vortex going on. One of the goals of this chakra is the redemption and harnessing of emotional wellbeing.

For those who feel there has been a halt, or stagnancy, in their sex lives—perhaps not feeling like having sex with their partner—it means it is stuck or dormant, but not gone.

You have not lost your drive, just lost touch with it. All you need is an awakening of the primal Self, as some women are calling it right now—a re-wilding. Why do we think Jesus was referred to as a lamb and a lion?

Yoga can do that.

Because of decades of untapped energy, I was in active combat with warring emotions. Now, my opened heart gifts me a healthy flow of feelings because I am anchored in safety and protection. This is emotional intelligence and health.

You can feel this way, too. You can speak your truth without being overly concerned about offending. You won't do it perfectly, but you can listen without judgment. It's the spiritual freedom that comes with surrender to the life that is larger, that is sourced in Creator. I extend this blessing over you, dear reader, a life that feels expansive. A life where being open to learning becomes your greatest joy.

Remember God's promise applies to you right now:

"Don't be afraid of things you might suffer. I will give you a crown of life."

REVELATION 2:10

If like me, you've had other Christians try to scare you about yoga's demonic roots, this is precisely why I speak my message; so that you can trust that your body resonates with the truth in every expression of faith: love, joy, peace, hope, kindness, and grace.

STAND ALONE

"May today there be peace within.
May you trust God that you are exactly where you are meant to be.
May you not forget the infinite possibilities that are born of faith.
May you use those gifts that you have received, and pass on the love that
has been given to you.
May you be content knowing you are a child of God.
Let this presence settle into your bones, and allow your soul the freedom
to sing, dance, praise and love.
It is there for each and every one of us."

TERESA OF ÁVILA, CHRISTIAN MYSTIC

I wonder, if for as long as you simply attempt to be a good person (versus a true, obedient one), you will not be pushed out of the nest to discover you are the woman who anointed His feet. She who sinned much was loved much; she who needed much was forgiven much (herein lies the power of repentance, of recognizing we can all admit the ways we've gotten caught up in our fears or unhealed nature).

This is a corollary truth of spiritual magnitude that cannot be over-emphasized. The shadow Self needs saving to be brought into the light. This is to diminish the hidden hold of a minimized story of letting me keep 'that' in the dark corner of the basement of my mind.

For there exists a realm where I'm a sinner, a tough cookie. Stubborn, a know it all. Moody, self-centered, entitled. She exists in chronos time.

God burned her up. Some call that realm hell, an age. It didn't last.

But me in *Him* in Kairos time? That's my infinite soul Self, a light-filled essence. That's the me that my great grandchildren will speak to in their hearts and feel my love flow directly to them from the great beyond.

Pull back the veil and feel the truth of Her. For in Christ is revealed the One Power, One Life since the dawn of time.

Speak this aloud: For we know that Christ loved (fill in your name) more than any other woman.

Sacral Story

Sacral chakra, as mentioned, represents the emotional connection to the soul.

In my own history, if I was going to save my marriage and my health, I'd need to pivot toward a life to be proud of. If I'm honest, I know there was a moment I knew my younger self would be mortified at the woman I'd become. I never imagined I'd create legacy out of illegitimacy.

Kneeling now, my intention to bleed truth, literally to be new wine poured out, means I'll have to move beyond any conditioned fear around the subject. I'll put on my breathing apparatus, helping me to breathe underwater (subconscious realm). Time to travel through potentially dangerous territory. The stormy seas of emotions.

The bastard daughter (me, Anita): I would be the one to break the pattern. I would be the one to hear God whisper that I was being a 'spiritual whore' and know exactly why and exactly how to shift.

Our energy is precious and needs to be guarded at times. We have had love poured into us by Creator. How we spread our love takes great discernment.

Not everyone should have access to your love and attention.

My golden retriever, Sierra, and I walked past the Adirondack chair on the front lawn of our South Jersey home. It was thirty degrees, a cold late-January day. I recalled the younger woman I was who desired to be free of sexual longing.

I can remember her wondering how a person keeps having sex with the same man for at least three or four more decades. I look back at that woman and know she was trapped in her fear, that she would succumb to her temptation to cheat. I want to tell her not to worry. I want to stroke her cheek and calm her.

I told her, do not focus on your weakness, nor the history of philandering and infidelity you inherited.

That is not *who you are*

I reminded her, generations before you created bastard children in the physical and spiritual realms, you will break the pattern.

You will set your great-grandchildren free

Young lover of union, I heard from inside, you will transform sexual energy into creative endeavors, learning the magic of alchemy. Your body will pray with Christ, your King, making you new, making your marriage bed new, too.

You'll learn to freshen what feels stale and lighten what feels heavy.

To save my marriage, I had to sacrifice. I had to walk away from friendships and group-thinking which brought me familiarity and comfort. I had a habitual way of seeing myself, operating as a flirt, a party girl, and an airhead. I was even given a nickname for my wild nature evidenced on the dance floor—Tribal.

For as long as I denied the obvious need to cut out my harmful antics, my body cried out in chronic pain, continued to binge drink, endured countless sleepless nights and unexplained trips to the ER for gastric distress.

I severed long held and deeply loved relationships (there is always sacrifice on the narrow road with Jesus)

I was convinced that they were the bad influence on me (an incredibly misdirected assumption). Little did I know, my pain body—my suffering Self—had been driving my life toward destruction, aka: trauma bonding. Blaming is a sign of our powerlessness.

Everything is happening for me, for my liberation

'Everything is happening for my freedom' became my new mantra. In this new world, I was no longer the victim. I would have to rise up higher. No more drama, or gossip. No more wasting of my precious gifts and energy. No longer would I be dividing up piles of blessings versus piles of curses. I kept stating that everything is included. I kept saying and feeling that I was fierce with reality.

I am fierce with reality.

For example, after that realization:

I was at a neighborhood gathering, and was pretty excited that things were moving forward with making this book a reality, so I began to give an update to a friend. After a few sentences, she found a way to sidle away from me, mid-story.

I didn't get to finish

I didn't go track her down. But, the next day, in my morning pages—words I write each morning for no one else other than myself, and for no other reason than to express the Self and ready for the day—I felt the upset rise from my heart. I began to cry. "I was talking, and you just walked away. I was sharing something important, and you just left me standing there in the kitchen, the smell of Bolognese wafting from the nearby stovetop." I wonder how many times we traded being heard for feeling safe as children?

These are the little heart remember-ings that are about our relation-ships and relating to others—the Sacral—that bubble up. With the help of expression, like morning pages, we don't carry disappoint-ment throughout the day. The repentance that arises when we realize the hours that turned into days, then weeks, as we were lost from the primal power of ourselves, gives way to the wisdom that all things are in constant flux, nothing stays the same.

Only this acknowledgment births the indestructible.

In reality, her leaving is all about her. It might be about her not following a dream. But it is not for me to decide what it is about. It is for me to only know her walking away was hers. My choosing to decide how to deal with it was mine.

It has nothing to do with me

In those moments, and in every moment of reflection, we must rely on the truth of the teaching: what we say is about us, but what someone hears us say is about them, and how they respond is always about them.

Conversely, our responses to others are always about ourselves.

This isn't a 'who did what to whom'. We've all done things like this. I wonder, in my heart of hearts, how many times I've done this to others.

I have digressed.

Sacral chakra is about relationships. So, what of the relationship between I and it?

We may think we're separate from all, and that which we looked at was 'out there'. We looked at 'it'. But truly there is no 'it'.

Every living and non-living thing is a part of us. If our response is anger, opinion, judgment, separation, fear or anything other than compassion, then we are not seeing from the heart/mind union.

When we make one big or small mistake, we often—because of the growing guilt in us—go on to repeat our conditioned poor behavior instead of repenting and admitting fault. Why? The simple answer—*fear*.

Our own voice judges us the most harshly. But that voice is simply a disconnected, abandoned little one, longing to be reunited with the inner family of you. Sound crazy? Perhaps explore how the voices of your past almost destroyed lots of good things in your life. Or examine how the voices of your past are eroding the good things yet to come in your life.

Guilt points us to reconciliation. It offers us a place to step off a destructive path and into salvation. We build ourselves a fire, stick by stick, and then enter into it and stand there—a living sacrifice. It is a sacred homecoming, in turning inward. All that is within us is destined eventually to be brought out from under the covers into the light. Renounce nothing. Ask to be shown all the skeletons. I had a dream about pink baby rats infesting the roots of our trees in the backyard but, come daylight (in the dream), they flew away as doves.

I will never lie to you

Giving up what feels comfortable can feel like intense grief and intolerable pain. Remember, a bad day for the ego is a celebration for the soul. You may believe there is a limited you—there is only a limited you when you think yourself to be limited.

What if we go through most of our adult lives merely tapping 50% of our full capacity because so much is hidden in the subconscious (remember, body is subconscious mind). What if it requires all your attention and commitment to seek the face of Christ.

What if nothing can die, ever?

What if the world really needs your fierce warrior?

Why present this so dramatically? Because we are dramatic in our actions. Because this narrow path includes engaging fully with the Good Friday phase, then the patient promise of Holy Saturday.

We cannot jump to Resurrection Sunday
any more than we can wish ourselves, with magical thinking,
into liberation.

It is in the loss, the shame, the fiery light of Christ's love, where He allows us to melt into His arms so that we might be remolded. Know that failure is always a gateway to transformation. For what human would conceive and consent to this mortification to be a part of God's divine plan for your life? You are going to have to keep showing up, serving, believing, praying, doing the messy work of your own sanctification. It's called practice for a reason. It won't look glamorous, but you'll be digging up the old, poisonous wells in Jesus' name. When you keep re-committing to simple disciplines done with love, you receive long-term benefits.

Alchemy, or transmuting our chakra 'demons', is the hero's journey to self trust. It leaves us to discover that abandonment of the Self is God abandonment.

And while we humans repeatedly break our own and one another's hearts, Jesus is not in that business. His steadfast love for us is what drags us out of the pit of depression. For all our devils will die or be loved to death.

"Evil is not immortal—Love is—And so are you!"

I COR 13, MIRROR BIBLE

To be balanced in the Sacral chakra, one would have healed any split between spirituality and sexuality. Historically, all religions have insisted on the necessity of healing a split from God but, while the world most certainly needs redemption, it's not a problem we fix by appeasing God. It's in the act of forgetting the truth. God's always been with us and on our side.

And guess what? It is often the church (any organized institution) that has created this unhealthy divide.

The chakra of sexuality and money issues (read: pleasure—greed or pauper mindset) is the place in the body that holds our misunderstanding of hidden aspects of the workings of the universe. On the surface, the world seems to operate on a plus/minus, failure/success, winner/loser system.

But in God's economy nothing is wasted, all is kindling. In a practical sense, we can face our issues in our tissues boldly, because our faith promises us that Jesus' sacrifice at the Cross covers all of our supposed sin. A grand reversal: He turns everything upside-down.

An authentic path toward truth in this kingdom leads downward… (Literally, look down right now. Isn't it odd that we are told in traditional verses to always look up?) A descent is more practical than an ascent. Because this is the direction the Cross would direct us—pain, mystery, mess, sex, sin, and family of origin.

Our illusions keep us from living as free men and women. Things are not as they seem. Physical reality is only a slim fragment of the entirety of the universe—our spiritual eyes open in stages. For example, what the heck are black holes anyway? Sorry didn't mean to send you off to google right there.

Whether it's an inner fantasy life, addiction to porn, sexting, or actual cheating, what this really points to is an excess of energy in this chakra. Every human wishes to be set free of 'dirty chunks of thinking', whether it is around sex or hatred, greed, or fear. Yoga is a way to still the mind so we might allow unhealthy, habituated thought-forms to burn up.

Despite our world being in an abnormal, fallen condition, we do not have to remain there. The universe is not governed by chaos and randomness. There is a web of interconnectivity called the quantum field. For just over 100 years, science has confirmed what yogis have known for thousands: interconnectivity in the known and unknown universe.

Grace is holding it all together for good. What we see and know in the physical realm is only the tip of the iceberg. The majority of the universe is invisible, dark energy and matter. You are primarily energy, and only five-percent matter. I like to imagine that all that dark energy and matter is comprised of the communion of saints—a collection of all those who have left this earth in human form and left with the purest energy of their souls

Make a list right here. Who have you loved that is now gone from their physical bodies? Who do you hope is not only watching with a smile but is included in the power of resurrected and eternal love from beyond?

Sacral chakra rules the watery emotions. Yes, E-motion as in energy in motion. When things are moving, nothing is really stuck. We were taught to control or avoid our emotions by people who wanted to control or avoid our emotions (and their own).

A conversation between my pastor and me:

Anita: When do you think, in evolutionary terms, the Soul was deposited into the creature?

Pastor: (he replied without skipping a beat) Now.

Anita: (taken aback with a woah!*) Yes, that's right. It's always now.*

My soul in Christ and my primal nature are meeting anew; like Christ being born amidst the barn animals, yoking creature and the creator. I can recall being in gorilla pose, hands under my feet, and hearing a soul message about this integration. Something like, "Oh, hello there, soul beast. Welcome to my being. You are wild and I need your nature to embrace the seductive and resplendent. We were never meant to be at war. Let's dance."

Maybe the soul is unconscious. It could be a beast like Sierra (my golden retriever) or an infant. Sierra doesn't know she gets dirty when out playing in the world. She gets mud on her belly and under her muzzle. She needs to be scrubbed behind her ears and doesn't enjoy it. But I am the conscious one. I can see that she needs to be cleaned. This doesn't make the dirt bad. It doesn't make the world bad.

Who was it who said you were naked?

There is often so much mud under my belly and on my muzzle. More and more, though, I feel more aware than Sierra, because we know we are creatures with consciousness, which makes us creators.

The rub is participation through prayer, community service, reading, chanting, yoga, meditation—participaction, really. I start my day with one of the boldest books I've found so far, *My Utmost For His*

Highest, Oswald Chambers. Paraphrased, he says, you want God to move or act?? Well, He's not going to.

You move. You act. Then you wait and watch.

> *"Put on your new nature and be renewed*
> *as you learn to know your Creator*
> *and become like him."*
>
> COL 3:10 NEW LIVING TRANSLATION

Honor your primal nature. Make shapes with the body to acknowledge it. Be respectful. Be expressive in the way of making sounds— grunts, howls—to allow it to be as it is. Shine a light on its primal needs for safety, food, procreation, pleasure, and connection.

STAND ALONE

I was awakened one day with these challenging words on the door-step of my heart. Yes, the harshness serves a high purpose but I have transcribed His words with fidelity… difficult, initially… maybe, but leaving you, respected reader, to interpret for yourself.

Smile, I imagine the Lord saying, then continuing: I have great news for you! You are all whores and you're all commissioned into the creation of the new Jerusalem. If you deny your whoredom, I will deny you.

Christ has chosen his bride and it's us—in all our messy, lusty, cheating, shadow-filled, greedy, lying ways; In our racist domination system and in our body chastisement.

We are meant to be uncomfortable with the above statement because we are meant to clearly see that, if we cannot include our own ridiculous attempts at worthiness, then the full power of the gospel cannot fulfill its mission.

For we still have a full measure of self-righteousness at work.

We've all been guilty of being promiscuous. But there is good news. Christ is the amalgamation of the divine and the human—we are 'wedded'.

As all energy is sourced in sexual energy, all are guilty of looking to the world and demanding: please me, love me, satisfy me, acknowledge me, comfort me.

There is a way to focus solely on God and what he's doing in your life so that you stay in your lane and develop inner healing power. The real bread of life. God always comes for the hungry and the thirsty and the desperate. If I have no needs, then He has no need for me.

Bring yourself into focus. In our having wed the world, we each might as well have emblazoned the scarlet letter on our heads and hearts.

Julian of Norwich's radical, optimistic theology gifted us the same message. She fully recognized human beings' carnal nature to screw God over, as well as one another. We expend an inordinate amount of precious energy attempting to proclaim our worthiness. And yet, Julian insists, "All will be well and all will be well and every kind of thing shall be well."

Take that in.

Not until we have demanded of Him—mirror in the sky—show
your face your power, your glory

As promised

Our weakness will unveil His strength

Our failure reveals the magnitude of His grace

Harvest my thoughts, Lord

You know how I've sown in my tears

When will I reap in joy?

No one comes to God perfectly

Nor do we consistently come in awe, wonder and gratitude

Not until we've first bloodied our knees

STAND ALONE

It is April 2020. My husband and I are inches apart on the living room couch, about to embark on a breath practice with world-renowned master Wim Hof, a 10-minute YouTube challenge to respiration, will (strength), and the nervous system.

My mind wanders. It is my Oma's birthday in heaven. She'd be a grand old 98, having died 21 years ago. Probably most interesting is that we're in the midst of the 21st century's first global pandemic, a modern-day plague—Coronavirus. We are being challenged to understand a new-to-us vocabulary: quarantine, shelter at home, Zoom meetings, health care heroes, and sacrifice for the common good.

My mind floats over to William Blake's words. The poet and mystic considered the unity of all men with each other and with the whole universe. In other words, I am my neighbor and my neighbor is me. All of the things that happen to any creature happens to the universe—all experiences are shared, collective, of humanity.

Blake refers to the Lord's Prayer, and the forgiveness of sins being the rule laid upon us by Christ in that prayer. Blake said that Satan's great function is to accuse the world of sin and, by abstaining from accusing anyone of anything, and forgiving all offenses, we can go beyond that negative by passing through it and leaving it behind.

While breathing into my belly, my thoughts stray: I am reminded of my having been persona non grata in our family... for so long. It's hard for me not to go all dramatic and make myself the victim. But no, I am on a path of accountability and, in that light, I shall tell you, dear reader, why that season—the longest and most painful one—was the place in time when God showed me the 'whys' of my sin and struggle. Whoever told you faith was a painkiller for suffering is a liar.

Our wound is the opening for the light to enter. Our ego inflation began as a protective measure for our hurting inner child. At some point we began to feed the bad wolf, this part of our Soul which has gotten lost and is on a rogue operation. We must find a way to bring her home. Integration. We know from Gen 2:7 that the soul is the result of the body (soul) and Spirit (life) joined.

I was reminded that, in the past, I had betrayed loved ones again and again with manipulation and gossip. It is absolutely mortifying to recall this behavior. Somehow, I had become an enemy of not just one but several people in my life. It would take years to explore this aspect of the Self. I spent ages living the question: am I bad at my core?

It turned out to be a really good question.

Jesus wants us to quickly move beyond the 'fall from grace' and enjoy being back in the garden with Him. If we insist upon our identity being rooted in bad behavior, we literally mock and reject Christ's sacrifice on our behalf.

Dear ones, I hope these practices help you pass right through that 'state' of sin. I hope you chip away at the scaly, surface layer. My sincerest desire is for these practices to allow God himself to draw you close and kiss all those boo-boos.

This is why, when I forgave my abuser, I was completely set free. One month before this book was due to be released, he came to me in my Spirit asking if I could finally let him love me, let him help me.

Through my teary overwhelm, I replied yes. Somehow, our enemy holds one of the keys to the gate of our Heaven. Jesus died for them, too.

What would happen if you began praying for your enemy right now?

Inhale this message: I want to bless my enemies.
Exhale this message: I give this desire to you, Oh God, because it often seems impossible.

There is a realm where we see all of humanity is worthy of God's love. Not a chosen few. We must find our way to discovering how we have objectified others even if not, in the same way, we were objectified, or we might find we are minimizing the ways we fall short. In my experience, to be far from God could be an inch or a thousand miles: this distance does not exist in spiritual terms. We are either 'in Christ' or have a need to repent/return. We don't want to find ourselves the older brother in the prodigal son story- on moral high ground.

I was saying to my 22-year-old daughter how I am not sure what people without a personal relationship with God do with their self-accusations.

But I do know—I remember well, just sitting in my murky mind unable to get beyond my own mess-making.

Then one day the gospel's power seemed to land in a way which no longer allowed any future attempts to make my being an imperfect human a problem. Suddenly, He showed me that I was in Him all along. To forge our identity, not from what we do in the world or even our relationships in it, is to allow our very worthiness to stem from an eternal connection. To the ego, this sounds entirely too ethereal. I

know this. I'm a wife, mother, writer, teacher, daughter, progressive…
a long list of how I might be introduced.

Once we confront the lies that success is rooted in digits after a dollar sign we challenge the narratives of capitalism, of democracy. We
challenge the idea that we are worth what we make. Or flip it—that
what we make could ever deliver our worth. A kamikaze yogi explores
this identity.

The power of true grace eradicates our personal anxieties that anything truly depends upon 'my' getting it right. Jesus keeps showing
up, announcing: "When will you get it? Your mess is mine."

To live 'from' the finished work of the cross
shifts our purpose and heightens our sense of responsibility.

If you are inspired by these words, that means He is doing it or did it
in you. If you are contemplating burning this book, well… I hope you
can sense me laughing… and still feel my love.

Because of our understanding from the Old Testament, we have
within us the false idea that we follow a God who sends plagues and
who loathes people because they do not adhere to His strict rules,
codes, and instructions. But then, when viewed through the lens of
Jesus, we realize this is just a world with all its wars, tsunamis, and
plagues just like there have always been. Jesus is our reminder that we
have access to God, right through our own hearts. No mediator, no
priest—the holy of holies is open for business. What do we get? His
Presence. The I AM announcing I AM always with you.

God in Jesus's image is the one who redeems the grief and doubt, not
the one who creates it. The physical horizontal realm, when intersected

by the vertical realm of Spirit, dawning from the East, will reveal more about the nature of God and reality. Think: Spirit unifies, ego divides. Ego isn't bad, it just isn't complete. And it is extremely frightened.

A Restless Soul

Most spring and summer mornings, I start my day by praying and relaxing in a weathered Adirondack that sits on my front lawn. My golden retriever, Sierra, always goes with me, lounging on the grass at my feet. I've got my freshly brewed coffee in hand and the view of green expanse in every direction instills peace, spaciousness, and delicious quiet. The oaks and poplars, dense with foliage, block our view of the river just beyond. Trees have been such a comfort to me in their steadfast witness of what God is revealing in the stillness.

Without fail, it isn't long before neighbors with their dogs begin walking past across the street. Sierra, at eleven years old, loves to make a ruckus by barking at them—it seems to have worsened as she's aged. I seem to have less patience for it than I did before. I begin by insisting she lie down, and I tell her to be quiet, stop barking, and be a good girl. She doesn't listen well, and tries to get up and continue to loudly express herself in order to be seen and heard by her doggie friends.

Each time this happens I have an inkling about what our embodied Soul is like and how she's teaching me something of value that I can share.

- The body likes discipline
- The body likes movement

- The body likes making sounds

- The body likes being seen and heard/witnessed

- The body is full of good energy

- This energy will express itself in harmful ways if not directed, harnessed, and transmuted for good

- The body and the Soul are intertwined

- The body appreciates grounding

- The senses are a precious gift to be appreciated and enjoyed

- The mind and the body are one organism

- The body will sacrifice its health for the psyche

- The body will sacrifice its comfort for the psyche

- The body is the revealer of truth, via tears, goosebumps, and chronic pain (Truth with a capital T)

- The body is an instrument which can be offered to the divine through yoga body prayer, dance, and other forms of authentic movement

- The Soul will become restless if not acknowledged as a lover of the arts, sex, and music

- If the Soul does not receive permission to enjoy what it was created for, the disconnect and block of shame will devour joy and pleasure

The 'barking body' will be a nuisance, and the body will be blamed for what is the responsibility of the conscious Self to enact—a life filled with the wonderful things God has offered us to enjoy freely.

When I get to the end of my life, I imagine God will ask me, "Did you enjoy it? Did you have fun and find a way to be in communion with my creation?

Perhaps he will continue and ask: "Did you get distracted, stuck in your head, worried about the past or the future—of which, neither place contains the pleasures and riches of the present?"

My Soul gets restless, but I've learned to listen to her persistent communication with me. I've learned that I can balance the mundane with the mountain-top experiences, and that my intimate partner within is the reason it all becomes a life of purpose, and I am deeply connected to the natural world. Our challenge is not only to tolerate the ordinary chores and boredom of life, but to engage with them from a place of presence, through curiosity and connection.

Those trees, this dog, the earth beneath my feet become companions on the journey, assuring me that I'm not alone; I'm seen and heard. My 'barking body' has a friend within who cares deeply about her sacrificial attempts at love.

You may be a Christ follower who feels like a foreigner in a world where divisiveness over topics is tearing apart governments and churches. You might have many friends who've given up on God and are seeking spiritual enrichment in yoga studios, and through Buddhist meditative practices. I am here to bear witness to the rich necessity of East meeting West. We can trust the guidance of the One leading us to try new things. Will you allow God to be as original with others as She is with you?

What I mean by that question is: maybe you are wired similarly to myself; I seem to fall easily into the trap that others' experiences of

God and mystery would have to stem from their practices instead of stemming from God and mystery.

Words get in the way—gnostic, heretic, esoteric, psychic, feminist, goddess, and pagan. Labels. All not helpful. Being in real, vulnerable relationships with real people who don't think like us is the way to humility and the way to form deep, rich bonds. Become the noticer of any judgment or ideas of separation. Be the one who frequently practices saying, "I can imagine why you feel that way. I hear you." This is an excellent way, without agreeing, to be more human and allow others to be heard.

Again, let us pause to acknowledge that this 'witness', this noticer, is always available, and we can allow ego to enter this space of non-duality, where fear takes a back seat.

Remember: if duality represents the opposites, then non-duality is like a deeper consciousness where there is a one-ness, calmness and flow of awareness without the fear of having to be involved in thinking there is one side or the other of an issue, situation, or thing. Paradox.

So while you're here—without waiting to the end of the section:

Bring your awareness to the back of your head, the spine, the seat, the ground—of you. It is as if you are pulled to the earth, because you are, by the giant magnet of gravity.

This action allows the 'front' of you, action of you, the speaker, to originate from the pause, the space, the Sabbath. When you do this, going about your business with awareness, you are allowing the Lord to lead.

It may appear to be such a simple thing: awareness to the back of the head, spine, seat, ground—being pulled to the earth by a giant magnet, but it can bring an instant and huge shift in you, therefore your actions, after doing this exercise.

The comments of what this felt like, from someone who had never done any body work or yoga, was that she felt a light connection (as in brightness), and then she felt the back part of her (shoulder blades and spine) was supporting /pushing the front part (chest stomach). When she stopped consciously doing the movement or pose, she felt that the energy continued operating behind the scenes to let the front half of her—her hands and arms—operate as if there were a superpower behind her.

We can learn from our neighbors and other spiritual practices, while remaining rooted in Christ. He is our firm foundation and we do not need to fear. Like the Israelites in exile in Babylon, we are called to be in the world, but not of it. We can love our neighbor as ourselves; we are to serve our communities with the Living Water which heals and energizes.

But too many Christians have depleted themselves.
They have not found inner peace.

We are told to serve and self-empty from our living Self until we are exhausted, when in actuality we have endless untapped 'death energy' ready to be expended. It's no wonder so many Jesus followers become burned out. They never learned how to go deeper and how to deeply rest, restoring and refueling. I believe the 'body disciplines' will restore us to the real power of Christ by bringing health to the body and peace to the mind.

A Sunday-only faith leaves Jesus impotent to help us heal and thrive the other six days.

Sacral Chakra Story

I was made in earnest, fascinated by the body, by death, and sex, and elimination. I have spent too much time wishing I were funnier, or could stay in the shallows longer. But I'll never forget that moment at a sexual being workshop. A young, gorgeous woman—pregnant and glowing—was asked to describe what she was passionate about (in a few words).

"Fucking and shitting," she replied.

My jaw dropped. My mouth hung wide open. I wished I had been so bold as to reply this way, for I, too, love and appreciate those two things. Without sex, none of us would be here—as well, what is life devoid of pleasure? And, without a good poop, we are all miserable.

And that, my friends, is a prime example of stating the great importance of first and second chakra health. Even our habitual pearl-clutching is an opportunity to awaken.

The incredibly evocative poet, Mary Oliver, advised us to 'let the soft animal of our body love what it loves'. We admire her words; we know they are true, but do we follow her advice? No, we are mostly mortified by our smells, sounds, and needs. We snuff out our hungers.

READ ALOUD
_____

an invitation

we are trapped

the world has our attention

and we have fallen prey to its lies about our own Souls

get busy

work for God, for the good

read the good book and all the dozens of words written
    about that book

pray in earnestness

with words, with kneeling, and with a script of thanksgiving

but I tell you

the Soul needs your full attention once in a while

a sabbath date would be ideal

do not delay the call of the wild

maybe to the Cooper riverside or the Schuylkill banks

a family of trees will do just fine

go there and enter

the time is anointed for your arriving

for your breathing in nature

your nature deciding to lean into the simplicity of Her

she has been preparing to reveal Glory back to you

through Christ may you see more clearly without the fog

may you hear more distinctly without the chatter

leave behind all the things you carry

come empty

come open

come curious

just come

alone

expecting the friend

to reveal something new

SPACE FOR MAKING SHAPES

Are you getting used to listening to your own voice? I bet it's wondrous and full of love. If you don't think so, you're not listening with your heart.

Repeat this phrase inside your mind or aloud:

This is my body, Lord, broken for you. Broken as in stretched. Broken as in feeling emotions. Broken as in submitted to be open and vitally alive.

Now, relax. Standing or sitting.

Inhale through your nose, then open your mouth wide and stick out your tongue.

Make the hahhhh sound. First make the sound softly, then let it grow louder. This is your lion's breath.

Let the exhale naturally join your voice.

Three times is a nice repeat for this one.

Return to a relaxed position.

Now let us take a posture in our body. Yoga teaches us that awareness and intelligence must infuse the body. Each part of the body literally has to be permeated by the intelligence. We must create a marriage between the awareness of the body and that of the mind.

Come to kneel for a yoga pose we call camel.

Kneel as if in prayer. Now make two fists. Bring your fists behind your back and rest on your lower back.

Begin to gently squeeze your shoulders together.

Inhale (imagine you are tilting your heart to the sky) through the nose, look up, then exhale (through the mouth or nose). Feel your knees steady.

Exhale and soften your face and jaw.

Inhale. You might feel your hips draw forward.

Exhale, empty of breath all the way to your toes. (use your imagination, face still toward the sky, maybe smiling.)

Now, lift yourself to be upright (hips were forward and your spine was arched)

Return to head, pelvis and knee in alignment, and reach your arms overhead, either through a forward or a side arm motion, pressing your palms in prayer.

Return them to your heart center by bending your elbows and bringing prayer hands in front of heart.

Pause, breathe… feel your palms pressing gently. Lunge one leg forward now foot flat, stretching the opposite front of hip. Steady now and feel . Stay a few breaths before switching. Come to sit or stand

Ask yourself: So, what's happening now?

Rest in child's pose for about ten breaths.

Child's pose reminder: seat to heels and rest head on pillow or block.

Next: a simple lotion practice. Grab your body lotion/cream. Open it and take note of the scent.

Now rub it into your hands and feel all the sensations.

Now, with a loving focus, apply it to your arms, hands, legs, belly, feet, and face. I know for me, when I get to my own pouchy belly, I have to say I love you even though you seem to keep getting bigger.

Although these practices may appear simple, even unimpressive, they have the power to transform the trajectory of an inherited, karmic wheel life.

SPACE FOR MAKING SENSE

Were you going to jot down a word or two on something you didn't
understand—something that you thought you would look up later?
Something you agreed with? Something you disagreed with? A word
you needed clarifying?

Was there something that came to mind about your own life and,
when you read part of this chapter, it reminded you to journal a bit
around it?

Here's the spot to jot those things down.

Writing Between the Chakras

If you can think back to the 'portrait' you may have done after the first
chakra section, can you repeat the sketch of yourself or that symbol
you chose? How will it be different now that you have more information about the whirling pools within you?

Can you love the emerging map of you?

What words resonated in this last section? Were you shocked by any?
Why?

SOLAR PLEXUS CHAKRA—THINK FIRE

The third chakra, the solar plexus, controls metabolism and digestion. Located about two inches above the navel, and known as the navel chakra, it often deals with raw emotions like anger and frustration. It is linked to our ability to manifest our inspirations and dreams. It makes sense that its element is fire and its color association is yellow.

The purpose of this chakra is to center us where the fire transmutes what needs to be healed. Here is where we burn our enslavements to comfort, food, sex. For we are wired for ecstatic bliss. Here's where our inability to feel 'noble' resides. Think: theology of energy.

The third chakra is will and power. When it is in excess, it looks to the world as an inflated ego—not a pretty sight.

We're being invited to will and power in partnership with the divine *power*. Note: power *with*, never power over.

The power in this chakra can be used for good when it is collaborative, when it builds others, and when it has an 'abundant universe' attitude. The beloved community is where all our gifts are shared.

The demon of this chakra, the solar plexus, aka manipura or lustrous gem, is shame.

How do you feel about the core of you? What does it mean? Is it solid or weak-willed? Do you feel different at certain times?

We are all—by virtue of being human—fairly weak-willed. Seriously, we are, by nature, challenged to start and stick with new healthy habits. This is mostly because of our negativity bias built into our brains which are made to keep us safe and the same. But Darwin told us those who can be most responsive to change will survive and thrive. It is our flexibility like a reed bending in the wind which will bring us to the other side of what we've deemed as failures of will.

Digestive issues are common when the solar plexus is out of balance. There are plenty of articles on chronic IBS being rooted in a stressful environment in which the nervous system was unregulated as a child—evidence that the stability of the nervous system is directly related to the quality/stability of the care and experiences received from parents/caregivers.

Work-life balance is important. If you do not honor your own needs, you will not be able to sustain that inner light. It is all well to serve others, but the Self must be cared for first in order to help others. Again, the practices help uncover stagnant, repressed energy.

How do you nurture yourself?

If you are a person who is born to serve, who takes great pleasure from serving, this service has to be balanced with not being a people pleaser. A huge percentage of the population do just that: please others at the cost of depleting themselves. This quality makes it difficult to open to receive God's love and blessings.

What does your will and energy look like? How about your passion(s)? Do you have an ongoing dialogue with a higher power—God. A check in? A reverence?

In your life, what if you lost all your clients, or your credentials, or your job? What would you be doing with your time? Would you feel worthy? Is that where you get your identity?

The third chakra is all about the core. Our physical core being digestion—an inner fire—and the core of us via inner resolve/strength. If you are having a hard time getting your day started—low energy— that points to your fire being dim. But you were born 'adamant'— from the first man, 'Adam', we have received the Zoe life of Yah Weh's love for humanity. So be *adamant* about your own health, your own journey. Allow the fire of the practices to build your diamond strength.

Healing the third chakra involves breathwork. Imagine fanning a small flame into a blazing fire for the purpose of burning down blocks to libido, desire, pleasure, and fun. I highly recommend YouTube videos with Iceman Wim Hof. His method involves three "pillars": cold therapy, breathing, and meditation It has similarities to Tibetan Tummo meditation and pranayama, both of which employ breathing technique.

Getting sunshine, eating all our colors, and feeling your emotions so as not to trap them, can all contribute to expanded energy. Discipline creates the container to store, tap in, and release energy—natural energy, not artificial energy from stimulants, like caffeine, which push the nervous system into stress. Your spine is an extension of your brain, your nervous system. I have provided many opportunities to make various simple shapes throughout but another mental note right here—daily move your spine in all 6 directions. Cat/cow, side to side, and twists.

It is better to tap into oneself and generate organic energy—to access the prana, or subtle energy, stored in the spine. Prana is considered a powerful force that flows through us—in Hindu tradition, prana, also called chi in the East, is sometimes described as originating from the sun, and connects all the elements or chakras. In Christianity, we might simply say the breath of Life. The goal is for the body to be in natural homeostasis.

READ ALOUD
_____

An Agent in Her Majesty's Service

meet Mary

holy Mary

mother of God

She dwells in you as an independent woman

simple vessel

earthen vessel

your faith causes you to conceive God as well

She's one of us

you are one of us too

He's one of us

and we are all

us

Solar Plexus Story

On Personal will/divine will: we need a cleansing fire.

Our doctors and nurses, on this spring day in 2020, are donning every form of protection over their orifices in order to block the first pandemic virus in our lifetime: COVID-19. They wouldn't even consider coming to work after a night of cleaning up their sick child's vomit without a hot shower, scrubbing under their nails, gargling, making every human attempt to remove the remains of sickness from their person.

A trash man wears his long-sleeved gloves and sturdy coveralls in order to best protect himself from the stench of garbage before returning home to make love to his young bride. Most certainly he would shower to get the actual day's work off of him.

I remember when my new friend, a prison warden, told me that the first thing he did when he arrived home after a day at work was to take a hot shower. In his own words: "Get the evil that exists there off me."

If only he'd known about third chakra transfiguration. I hope he reads this book and contemplates the mirroring of our divine nature as seen in Jesus.

Our own tradition refers to our pain body as original sin, and yet we have not been given sufficiently powerful tools for transforming and becoming a rare, new breed of human. Not only do we carry in our cells the unresolved struggles of our ancestors, but we add to that our own unprocessed emotions from this life.

We are walking around covered in dense, dull, dead energy, but know little about how to get cleansed. Let us explore micro-moments of real peace.

We are called to participate by using all our tools, battling in the Spirit realm with our physical and visible breath-body.

"What blind guides! Nitpickers!
You will spoon out a gnat from your drink,

yet at the same time you've gulped down a camel without realizing it.
Great sorrow awaits you religious scholars and Pharisees—
frauds and imposters. You are like one who will only wipe clean
the outside of a cup or bowl, leaving the inside filthy.
You are foolish to ignore the greed and self-indulgence
that live like germs within you.
You are blind and deaf to your evil.
Shouldn't the one who cleans the outside also be concerned
with cleaning the inside? You need to have more than
clean dishes;
you need clean hearts."

MATTHEW 23:24-26 THE PASSION TRANSLATION

The chakras we've worked on so far are now primed to combine and supply the energy we can use to create personal power. Learning how to activate our own will, in conjunction with being in Christ, produces transformation from primal instincts. Your Holy Spirit quickening will help you realize every part of you was created to glorify your bridegroom. Love is eliminating fear. And when we eliminate fear, we abolish the 'reptilian complex' rooted in our amygdala which births the divine instincts of love and compassion to rule our actions in this world.

Philosopher, Georg Wilhelm Hegel said:

> *"Thus to be independent of public opinion*
> *is the first formal condition of achieving anything great."*

What does it mean to be transfigured? It means the inner matches the outer—by virtue of showing the world my messy insides—the world being: my people, my community, my family—they see theirs, and oftentimes they hate that. But I've gotten stronger because I see the truth; it's become my superpower to keep showing the world that messy insides are glorious.

The third chakra's element is fire because it is busily burning up the unhelpful habits and ideas we have about our inherited transgressions, our sexuality, and our difficulties in personal relationships.

You know how easy it is to get distracted from the work you are here to do. For example, I start my day wanting to tell some men in 'power' what I think about how judgmental and critical Christians can be, how we must guard against this hypocrisy. At one point, I would have sent a critiquing text but, after praying and dancing, I am relieved of any responsibility to criticize, to be right, to share my thoughts from that platform of righteousness. I am assured that my being in the local body of Christ is sufficient to get this message across.

On the day I was writing this section, I was in a group text with some ladies. They were sharing pictures of themselves—selfies—and I don't think one person 'liked' or 'loved' my picture. I am crying as I write this. I cried when I realized it then, too. I could easily have dropped into self-pity and created a 'story' in my head about why that happened—perhaps I have given you the impression that I did fall into that pity pit. I kept teetering, on the edge of doing so. But then I allowed the emotion, the genuine sadness, to flow through me because I was able to see that I was disconnected from the group. There was nothing for me to do about it then, or today. Today I am charged with writing this important chapter on how you, dear reader, can find power in my examples and create your own focus on reparenting through a connection to the Father. I am certain the circumstances triggered those tears in the now to heal an old story from adolescence.

So, on that day, I put on Rihanna's *Love On The Brain*, and I danced a bit. During this brief respite, I began smiling with the inner knowing that, because of my love for Jesus, He too has love on the brain for me. I was then, and am continuing to enter the divine mirror aspect of our intimate relationship. The world will always be filled with disappointment and distraction; we are responsible for continuing to claim energies available to us from our shadow, our inner masculine and feminine dancing, the collective unconscious, and even archetypal energies like Mary Magdalene, the one Jesus loved best.

For a season, the inner energies of me were expanding into the upper spiritual chakra realms and I began to lose my sense of Self and purpose. It is difficult to describe, but I was feeling too amorphous, too archetypal, and not Anita enough. I am so grateful that my pastor, and my husband, kept pointing me back to being Anita, and how she is God's purpose. Here is another example of how being in community is important for our own transfiguration.

> *There is such a huge difference between*
> *window-shopping and mirror-gazing; one condemns the other transforms.*
>
> FRANCOIS DUTOIT, MIRROR BIBLE

To remain honest in the flesh and deceitful in the Spirit is to live untransfigured. An inability to be fully autonomous sounds like a heart heavy with blaming. This immediately points us to having given away our power. Victim mode—I think we are all guilty at times. Take a moment here and record the last time you blamed someone else for causing you unhappiness or discomfort.

Your words are not in alignment with your thoughts because you do not sit in your seat of personal power where who you are is fueled by the Spirit who made you. Not sinning out of fear limits your capacity to individuate and grow in sanctification. Operating from the secure, grounded place of being loved allows us to be fully human—imperfect, sometimes wrong, and less judgmental of our fallen nature.

The lower two chakras in the first half of life allow us to merge with group-think and feel comfortable that we fit in with our people, but when we enter our 30's and 40's we begin to discern what is offensive to our own soul. This is the path of individuation and will birth in us the joy of being comfortable in our skin, announcing:

I love how I am made! Maybe quirky or more serious some days,
it's a privilege to explore all the hidden aspects of being me.

The absolute earth of you—your body in density—remains, yet somehow you are lighter. You carry yourself differently because you carry the Friend differently. Your resurrection body is emerging.

> *"We can manifest a physical body that is*
> *free of the tyranny of the genes we inherited from our parents*
> *and the medical maladies they bring us.*
> *But even more important,*
> *we can unchain ourselves*
> *from the limited emotional and spiritual stories we inherited*
> *or bought into during the course of our lives."*
>
> ALBERTO VILLOLDO, PH.D., MEDICAL ANTHROPOLOGIST

Sometimes you carry Him as a babe in your 'womb' center. You imagine him growing and bouncing around, playful, happy to be home in you. Afterall He is our Son! Sometimes He is you, though. You are aware of your inner child being the replica of you and in need of your attention and care now. In the present you are given many opportunities to re-parent the unmet needs of your inner child. As you gaze at a baby or toddler, this unexpected feeling bubbles up, bringing tears of recognition that, indeed, she is here, feeling loved. Some teachers of re-parenting use the idea of imagining you have an inner foster child, more a stranger. I like this, and would add that he, too, is in Christ.

One simple way to see how we do not honor our own life force is that if we imagine we are driving with a real child in the car—if you've ever placed a child in your car (and are not used to shuttling children around) it is quite a new feeling of responsibility and awe. If we imagine we are driving with ourselves, a child, in a car, we would take the extra care that we do not presently afford our own inner child Self. Say right now aloud—I will save you.

Jung called the soul voice the ego conscious of the Self.

Your ego is being molded by the hands of the Potter;
some days you swing wide to feeling the fullness and completeness
then you can be assured you will swing in the other direction-
emptied and lost,
humbled and searching.

Eventually, the energies will balance and you will rest
knowing illumination is at the core of you.

In my own journey, sometimes I feel I am being reborn, and other times I know I am being made from the remains of the rubble of my former Self; all the ways I questioned my abilities and my failures, my

serious concern for my memory, despising my own 'broken mind' and
difficulty in creating in a linear format with focus and attention.

*"What do you mean?" exclaimed Nicodemus. "How can an old man go
back into his mother's womb and be born again?"*

JOHN 3:4 NLT.

I think, to be back in the womb, to be carried and nurtured by the
Father who I imagine to be a brown-skinned Mama, is to let the
Spirit surround us again. I think that if Mary was good enough to be
God's mom, She can be ours too. We are led by the winds of life to
explore and love and serve, to enjoy the safety of being inside Christ's
womb-heart.

No one can harm us there.

We are buffered in layers of warm, protective covering.

Can you imagine placing yourself back inside the dark, quiet, welcoming space of the Mama's heart. Might you sit on the floor of your
dimly-lit closet and take some breaths?

Going into the OT, we read:

*You are unmindful of the Rock that bore you,
and you forgot the God who gave you birth*

DEUT. 32:18 NIV

We might climb down into God's womb, but will we hesitate because
we worry God might not be patient, might not absorb us for the time
it takes us to get still?

Refreshed, rested, and transformed, we re-enter the world carrying a newly sparked inner light, forged in our submission to 'simply be'. We now embody Psalm 23. *"She restores my soul."*

Have you seen the movie 'Up'? There is a scene where the dog is distracted every few seconds by the squirrel… that's basically been me for two decades. Earlier in the book I mentioned adult ADHD. It is much more prevalent than I realized.

My mind in Christ means I can do tasks that the old me could never have dreamed doing. This is the chakra which assures we say 'yes' to the movement from being slaves of God to being friends. We are not just following rules; we trust ourselves to discern, to pray, to wait, to build with others, to believe that He wants to see us free. In this chakra we stay aware of any tendency to be willful, to be rebellious for rebellion's sake. I must check myself daily. This is why I spend a lot of time yielding on my knees, because I know that my immature ways could resurface if I'm not conscious.

And so it is through this sense of having a will that we engage our future Self.

At the end of this section—or skip ahead now to the space provided, or grab some extra paper—take a few moments to journal about a scenario you would like to see yourself enjoy.

During more than two active years of writing, I would future-self journal (a term coined by The Holistic Psychologist) about the book tour, chanting the names of God with my readers, seeing people receive clarity about divine practices and love, and having my mom proudly by my side. By virtue of our loving God, we are wired to dream big.

The demon of shame is projected on us from the outside and causes us to live in a state of 'something is wrong with me'. Maybe at any moment everyone is going to find out. Up until recently, if I received a message or a text: 'can I talk to you?', my body immediately went into flushed shame mode, and then the thought would pop in: uh oh, what did I do wrong now? Seriously…

I've since discovered a lot of us do that.

My power kept arising in me as I dared to take small risks daily. I would force myself to read something aloud on Instagram, or make a meme that was 'kinda out there' and post it, knowing I understood what I was trying to say, but others would think I was weird. And then I began to notice the synchronicities, the more I did, the braver I was—the more life enchanted me.

What might one of these small risks be for you?

Maybe text someone something right now—allow yourself to be vulnerable. Know that you might be ignored or viewed as too much at times. Know that you will survive this 'test' and grow stronger as you let go of a desired outcome.

This center of you is a crucible of your transformation. Holocaust survivor Viktor Frankl said, "For what is to give Light must endure burning". Know there will be people who ostracize or fear you for your individuality. As a Jesus loving Yogi, my first five years were a series of rejections, worried letters from concerned family members— even being preached at from the pulpit of a large church on Easter Sunday not to treat faith as a smorgasbord where one could choose from Buddhism and yoga, but to only eat from the Jesus bread.

Anger that is synthesized is incredible fuel from which to create; not from an 'I'll show you' resentment, but from a place of more truth in love. We must give ourselves permission to say there is much to be angry about. We must give ourselves permission to find our agency and inner authority.

That's just one example. I have mined a shit-ton of anger to place in my crucible. All our shadow aspects make for excellent material in the fire of manipura. This is why my inherent rebel nature purifies into being an ideal partner to history's greatest rebel of all—Jesus. Which is Him, which is me? It matters not. The world needs us to build a raging fire within, in order to burn up the trash we have accumulated. Say aloud-I burn the trash in me in an attempt to reduce suffering in our world.

> *How else do we expect the living waters to flow from our 'belly'*
> *as He promised?*
>
> JOHN 7:38

Scientists are now discovering that the gut/the belly, plays a critical role in the emotional life of a person. The gut, also called the enteric nervous system, has many nerve cells which create a 'brain'. Studies show it can react or 'think' independently of the brain in our head. This is why we have a 'gut feeling' about something, or a 'gut reaction', or why we get an upset stomach when we are afraid or anxious. Without strength and courage burning in our belly, our faith walk is weak-kneed and lily-livered.

Looking outward incessantly for validation, needing to be right, to be the one in the relationship holding the worldly power, comes from an insecure root.

Jehovah Jireh, I know I radiate power sourced in your divine strength.
Power with, never power over.
Embolden us to take a look at what's been passed down to us.

The Buddhist teacher, Pema Chodron, reminds us that, rather than letting negativity get the better of us, we can acknowledge, in the moment, that we feel like shit. She asks us not to be squeamish about taking a thorough look at our own shit.

There is fertilizer for your growth. Plant a single seed—a prayer—and allow the Logos, the logic of your life, and your practices to water it. You'll be amazed.

I see people everywhere: empaths who feel the world's pain and take it on as their own until they break from the weight, repeating childhood patterns until either they get sick or finally break the chain that they are not the world's savior.

This is the gospel good news of the power of knowing Christ personally. Our connection to the Spirit realm, where Abba dwells, fills us with the parental love we didn't get, the parental attention we so desperately needed. We get it now. It flows as new energy to our seed of an inner child, watering her. Today you begin your rescue mission—a sweet reunion with your inner child. Bravo.

SPACE FOR MAKING SHAPES

Get ready to hear your own voice take you through movement. Grab that phone and record the following. Then play it back for growth on more than one level.

Practice uniting what appears to be opposites.

The shape of the Cross already shows us the truth of reality: mind and body, East and West already unified.

"He who seeks vengeance must dig two graves,
one for his enemy, one for himself."

CONFUCIAN PROVERB

Who do you hate? Fear? What makes you suspicious? Be honest… let your heart speak.

In Christ, God loves the whole world now. May we pray with our body in order to bring peace into our hearts and minds; letting go of our fear, stress and need for control.

Stand now and bring your prayer hands to press at heart center.

Close your eyes.
Breathe naturally.
Reach your arms over head and clasp your hands, turning the palms up now.
Stretch to the right side, relaxing the shoulders, smiling.

Then after a few breaths go left, feeling your feet steady.

Come to center and, as you lower your arms, roll out your wrists.

Stand firm and steady in mountain pose now.

It might feel like you're just standing there, but mountain pose—tadasana (tah-DAHS-uh-nuh)—is an active pose. It helps improve posture, balance, and brings a calm focus. Never underestimate the power of the pause.

Its name comes from the Sanskrit 'tada' (meaning 'mountain') say that now—*tada*!!! as if to say—"Here I stand. Tall. Silent. Still. Witness."

Asana (means pose). Tadasana is the foundational pose for all standing yoga postures. Being steadfast in nature is foundational in all of life.

Notice your feet, feel your spine straighten, and imagine growing taller through the crown of your head.

In mountain, we bring ourselves to a posture of waiting.

Now roll your shoulders around—forward a few times then back.

Exhale loudly.

Reach arms back up and press palms together, overhead, then return them to the heart.

Bring one hand on belly and one hand on heart.

Take five deep belly breaths, puffing it out like a balloon.

Now bring one hand on forehead and one hand on heart.

Take five deep breaths—be aware that your lungs are filling up too all the way to the back (not just the belly).

Then reach arms wide, spreading fingers, and look up.

Feel your shoulders drawing together.

Say aloud: My heart is open and I have faith in you, Oh Lord.

Stand in mountain for a few breaths- feet steady, belly button gently engaged to protect the low back, heart slightly lifted and then: end by shaking and even jumping—shake your hands, arms, and legs in an effort to let go of any final bits of resistance to being love in the world.

Later

Engaging your imagination—put on some calm music and make yourself something delicious and nutritious—meal or snack. When we first learned to cook food, we became truly human. How distant we are from connecting the dots from the source to our plate.

So now, be mindful of the music, the smells, the textures, the colors of the food.

When I go back to childhood and recall my Oma cooking for us, I think of pierogis, stuffed cabbage, potato pancakes and mushroom soup from the can. My Oma also baked incredible tortes and cakes! But she didn't teach me. As much as she loved me, I wasn't permitted to be in the kitchen learning from her. Writing that makes me well up a bit. I lost the connection because she lived under near constant stress. I have restored it with my own young adult children, however.

Can you bring to mind an adult preparing food for you? What smells and meals come to mind?

Be present. Let's connect those dots now.

Sit alone to nourish your soul.

You could either imagine feeding your inner child, your orphaned, anxious energy or feeding Jesus. This is fixing your gaze on things that cannot be seen.

Close your eyes and pay attention to the temperature of the food if you cooked it.

Be hyper aware of the taste. Use words to describe the food as you chew.

Engage in a relationship with your 'child' or Jesus, being silly and saying things like: How do you like it? I made it especially for you! Is it too hot, honey? Too spicy? I hope you feel nourished.

I love you and I love making you feel special and relaxed, filled up with goodness. Give thanks for all the hands along the way who helped you experience this sacred returning to food as holy; food beyond filling the belly. Satiating at a whole new level.

Our cruciform faith ensures that we go wide in the Spirit, bold and stretching, but then return deep into truth- fully human is the hardest and most worthy endeavor.

> *"Why do we need to commit to one path?*
> *You cannot create a map to somewhere you've never been*
> *by using various pieces of other maps"*

CHRISTOPHER WALLIS, TANTRIK YOGA TEACHER

More Movement and Practice

There are crosses we are meant to shoulder with Christ, but many burdens we can roll back to God. Let us engage our imaginations again.

Identify one of your burdens right now.

Place it in an imaginary bowling ball that is at your feet.

Crouch down.

Roll it to him. Let it go away from you.

Wait… pause, breathe…see if he rolls it back

SPACE FOR MAKING SENSE

You know what to do here. Go for it. Throw yourself completely into it.

Writing Between the Chakras

Want to revisit your view of yourself again? Without looking at your previous sketches, if you did them, can you create an image of yourself here? Can you mark the chakras (we've covered so far) on your illustration?

THE HEART CHAKRA—THINK MARRIAGE

The fourth chakra is heart. Its location is obvious given its name. Its color is green, as in 'ever' green. The element associated with the heart is air. To live from the heart untainted is to trust Christ's life in you. This original goodness was mastered in the person of Jesus, in Him being the Lamb. His heart's eye sees clearly, is uncontaminated by memory or desire. In your soul, you are married to Him, you: man or woman, are the bride being led into a mesmerizing dance. Your carnal mind cannot fathom but your spirit mind knows. Breathe in, breathe out. Faith that arrives by Spirit is deeper than knowledge that arrives by the word or letter of law.

When I asked myself how to introduce this section, I knocked on my heart a few times, took a lion's breath, then said, "Jesus, show me to me, show me the relationship I have with my own heart, letting go of everyone else and resting in my enough-ness to listen to the one true voice within."

May you feel the love right now through the eyes of your heart that Jesus promises. Whether it comes through as Him or your own loved ones, you are no different than me, for this opened up as I practiced unifying my mind, body, and breath.

You, lovely reader, were made to trust your own connection to God, the divine source of all. You were made capable of tuning out the world's noise so that your soul knows you have shown up in earnest. This is how our Christian tradition began centuries ago, and yet the 'detour' away from simplicity has caused so much lostness, even violence. Your divine spark increases as you change your relationship to your breath, the Ruach. You will discover not just renewed energy, healing and clarity—you will discover *power*.

Your heart, all broken, lost, and armored, is worthy of your efforts to repair it and release the past. *Inhale future you, exhale former you.* See how in the *now* you are okay? Every 'now' that follows asks you to remember this feeling—of future-ness and clean-slated-ness and you-purity. Your heart knows you. Will you let it know the truth? Will you allow it to experience the fullness of your commitment to self-knowledge, beyond head belief?

The heart chakra journey will ask everything of you; challenge you to the core of identifying what real is, what protection is, to discern between conditioning and inheritance. The heart chakra journey will support letting go of what's already dead, and releasing all the 'could have been' and 'should have been' stories.

The heart chakra includes the lungs, which are often clogged with grief. A broken heart. Divorce, death, abuse, all fit into this dark side of the heart and draw its energy away from compassion and vitality. Physically, this relates to circulation, asthma, and tension between the shoulder blades.

If you genuinely want to witness the heart as evergreen, you'll view the trees releasing their leaves without fanfare, and recognize how you, too, can keep letting go.

READ ALOUD

It's okay. It's only you. Stand, open your mouth, open your heart, participate.

Little Drummer Girl

I lift my drum out of my chest in the wee hours of the still yet
    darkened morning

tap tap tap
awaken little drum

me and my drum
we become one in the promise

honor with glory
honor with praise

I lift my drum out of my chest in the wee hours of the still yet
    darkened morning

tap tap tap
such a powerful drum is this!

me and my drum
we sound the alarm
turn back!
Heart drum
drum beat
strumming

embrace the *love* for it has been flowing
in your blood since
the dawn of time
embrace Love's power
it has been saving you
since the first burst of light cast out the darkness

me and my drum
we are thrumming a new ancient song
alpha the Christ is your signature
omega with Jesus
you are seated in Papa's lap
tap tap tap
tap tap tap
ba dumpa dum dum

Chakra Story: Seeing With the Eyes of the Heart

One time I saw my aging face in the up-close car reverse mirror and was horrified, only to admonish myself. At that time, 'someone' inside me began to cry. I found myself apologizing to her. "Oh, honey. I'm sorry. I didn't mean to hurt you. I love you, and you are perfect in your wrinkles and no-makeup, simple face." When that happened, that time, I felt better for talking to the inner-me. She needed me to, and I began to stop my chronic self-abandonment.

To see your body from the inside of your heart is to look through the lens of love; to not ignore imperfections and pain. It is to be compassionate. As you become more aware of your body and its parts, you will be asked to sit with the judgments: overweight, wrinkles, saggy skin, small breasts, short legs, big nose, crooked teeth. There is so much to unpack as we come into a new relationship with our body's shortcomings—not just shortcomings, we could be dealing with chronic pain or disability. This acceptance points to our wounds with the feminine and the mother aspects of God.

STAND ALONE

Anahata—Unstruck

I have developed an open, tender heart, one that is anchored in safety. It is spacious and allows endless love to flow through without becoming depleted. Where once there was shame from near-constant offense, I have become unoffendable in a world bent on stealing our peace.

I want to invite you to recall the last time you found yourself in a conversation with someone or a group, and either you were at a loss for words in the way of being a fish out of water, or you were simply spewing words, mostly meaningless or, occasionally, sharp and cutting.

Can you identify if, after, you were filled with shame? You might have asked yourself back then: what is wrong with me? Why am I so awkward? Why do I not know the appropriate things to say? Why do I interrupt incessantly to get my thoughts across—thoughts which are not worthwhile. Empty words. Do I have an empty heart? What of this mind? Why do others seem to be at ease in themselves?

This was my life. I was always the one who opened mouth to insert foot. Then I was embarrassed. Did I have no original thoughts? Why couldn't I seem to wait patiently until a person was finished before I butted in? Too much talking is a sign of unprocessed anger.

Were these qualities going to doom me to a life of feeling confused about why relationships felt so difficult and complicated? I would come to realize they'd been created from an old wound, not from a whole woman but a desperate scrap of one.

When you live from your unstruck heart, you are vulnerable, and show the world the you that was hidden (even from yourself) for so long—it is supremely brave and incredibly liberating.

Every human internalizes experiences we were unable to process at the time, and so the body—your hero—has stored it in your cells. Your mind/body is always working hard to keep you safe. Rewiring the brain is one way to heal and address the inner emotional and energetic landscape. We have entered a new paradigm where we advocate our own healing and take accountability for the ways we can incorporate wellness practices, addressing all our parts: mind, body, Spirit, ego, inner child, and soul. I recommend the new book *Cured: the Life Changing Science of Spontaneous Healing* by J.Rediger, M.D.

Finally, crucial questions formed from this catalyst: I have lots of close friends, so why doesn't anyone ever turn to me to share their deepest heart, their struggles? Am I incapable of really listening with an open heart? Do I not have within me a shred of compassion to witness with?

At thirty-eight, I found myself at a small, local yoga studio searching for the lost contents of my heart. Would these yogis be more likely to help me than the Jesus followers at churches I had previously attended? There was something here with these yogis that I did not sense in those churches—an earnestness of presence, a dedication to discipline, a sincerity of vulnerability, and no fear of being seen.

Initially, I didn't fit in—oh, that was for certain. For starters, I had an extremely hard time understanding all the unfamiliar terms. There I was, on the mat, an almost-forty-year-old-woman, with low emotional maturity and self-awareness. I would have to adopt a beginner's mind and be less judgmental of myself. If only we could trust…

Emotional maturity is a revolution of *evolution*

I wondered if I was capable of true compassion, even empathy. I suspected I was numb. I had no idea from what, but I didn't seem to be able to tap into anything except envy, anger, frustration, impatience, and judgment. It was almost scary how those feelings came naturally. Am I good or not? At the core of me, I needed to know of what essence I was comprised. Am I simply a carnal-minded physical being enslaved to duality or am I born of the Spirit? Subconsciously, I'd been comparing myself to my husband for a decade—he's the good one, the angel. I am the troublemaker, problem child, the one in need of repentance. My rebellious nature was on everyone's nerves.

Desperate now, I would begin to live the question of my own goodness.

Over time, I discovered:
consciousness
grounding
presence
Spirit/Unity
heart opening
living with intention
chakras
energy body
somatics
nervous system regulation
polyvagal theory

Adult survivors of all forms of abuse, including insufficient parental bonding and disordered attachment, are often living with the feeling that their bodies are no longer safe to dwell in. Their existence is primarily an affair of unhealthy, habituated, and conditioned thinking. For those adults, for neurological safety, a protection is formed over the heart, often called armor. When that happens, no adult wants to rip off that layer of protection. It serves a purpose. But it is not meant to continue to harden like thickening ice.

Removing this layer is achievable through self-work and the practices in this book. They will open us to pure vitality as we feel true grief, true anger, true self-compassion. Check in right here, reader—do you desire to feel more?

Does that seem like a quality you'd like to emerge?

Would you like to engage with, and embody, an emotional self you can express and trust?

> *Her mouth speaks from that which fills her heart*
>
> LUKE 6:45

In my experience, Jesus has been the divine gaze, the attunement we need to heal our attachment childhood wounding.

The Torments of Grief and Envy

Through genuine expressions of grief, we can reconnect to our true Self. Up until last year, when our Godson Kyle died of a brain tumor, I had only grieved my Oma who was like a second mother and sister to me. For the better part of my childhood, Oma and I shared a small bedroom in our row home.

Some people I know are dealing with unimaginable losses.

My grief patterns have come from the ending of so many friendships. An awful pattern I found myself repeating. Loss is loss. Grieving is grieving. It might be that you have lost loved ones, severed friendships, or perhaps are grieving the end of a marriage. Even agonizing over a loved one going to prison.

Our first Self, the one we've hidden from our whole lives, is one we've labeled with a sticker called *fear*. Yet, Jesus takes our idea of separation from Him and sacrifices Himself to end that very idea. That first Self is one that we have been led to believe is just too weird, too honest or too emotional.

I am too _____

Lovely reader, fill in the blank.
Everyone has the thought that they are 'too' something.

When our son left for college, we entered the empty nest stage. The month before his departure, I began to notice a painful, tight, and heavy sensation around my heart. This was the beginning of a rising awareness of this energy center's awakening due to the building of grief around this massive shift in how I was needed as his mom.

I can now gauge how to shift my energy in order to regulate (breath work, time in nature, a massage, acupuncture, stretching, telling Jesus I need help identifying what's happening in my body) when belly bloat and heart heaviness set in.

The heart center is where union of the inner sacred masculine and feminine dance. In psychology, the terms are animus and anima. No matter your physical gender, we all have both aspects operating in us and, from a scriptural perspective, we humans are always the 'woman' in the bible story. It is about humanity being the bride of Christ. Think about that, men. I can imagine you putting on a dress to embrace feeling pretty for your King. To overcome society's judgment around this attempt to break free. You are Mary Magdalene, you are Mother Mary, you are the container, the womb heart/the garden for Jesus to dwell in and grow like a seed.

To open the eyes of the heart is to have a more fearless and inclusive view of the Self and humanity. This is the path to living a life that is unoffendable. Can you imagine that? I know I could not have—I seemed to live in a near-constant state of offense. My family would remark about mom's rude comments to the innocent sales clerks behind counters. Yes, me, projecting anger I could not handle. *But the opposite of love is not rage, it is indifference,* says Valerie Kaur, activist, documentary filmmaker, lawyer, educator, and Sikh faith leader.

We can be so anchored in our deepest, truest, safest heart womb, that no matter how the world treats us, we are immovable. This is not to say we accept poor treatment. We do not. We discern what is worthy of a response from our agency, our inner authority, about what each of us will stand for.

We don't know what we don't know. We cannot see: we are blind to so much in our shadow, our subconscious. One day we find curiosity growing, while judgment diminishes—a heart pivot in the direction of compassion and forgiveness.

I had defined my worth in sexual terms for so long. Christian author Jen Hatmaker has a series called *White Women's Toxic Tears* on Instagram. She partners with Pastor Lisa Sharon Harper, a Black woman, in order to call out the many ways that whites are both inordinately fragile and manipulative with our skin color supremacy. She touches on the patterns of our damsel in distress, our using femininity to get us out of trouble with our traffic tickets. It is commonplace and time to bring awareness to how we are behaving as if we have no power—because, in an earthly sense, we often do not have power in arenas of business and politics ruled by old, white men. But in a spiritual sense, we have all the power we need.

I had no idea this was a common sign of unhealed sexual trauma. I realized the abuse I had endured instilled a false belief that my body was more valuable than my mind and my heart. Fear seemed so at home, cozy in its corner of the heart. Settled, seemingly unpacked there for the long haul. In my case, I never knew there was a brave, new heart waiting to be transplanted.

… A brave, new heart with my name on it. A fair trade—a stone for flesh.

Simply bringing the light of awareness to the body-disconnect delivers healing psychic-soul-energy.

Take Einstein's theory of relativity, which is commonly known as $E=mc^2$. The 'm' as the matter of you, the physical part you can touch. The c squared, in my understanding, is a multiplied powerful awareness—light—on which we focus. For example, that flexed thigh muscle. This combination equals a new E. Energy as a healing force. An expansion. Wow, dear reader, what could that 'c' be for you: cosmic, consciousness, Christ?

Forgiveness is the primary healer of the rejected, grieving heart. First and foremost self-forgiveness. We allow our own guilt to create a sticky layer, on top of which all other offense lands and makes its home; a thickening layer of armor.

Take a few moments this week and write down the names of anyone you may harbor resentment, anger, and hardness toward, asking God to show you next steps in your full healing and heart softening.

READ ALOUD

How often will I let my Jesus
climb up on his cross
allowing the one I knew to die again
allowing the one I don't recognize to rise

to sit in the throne of the Heart is to sit with truth
to let the flames consume all that is not truth
this is not for the faint of Heart
no, one must have on their mind of Christ
a level of self-trust equaling God-trust
self-love a superior signal to God love
for God love is the steppingstone to self-love
one 'seeming' so much more accessible and divine than the other

SPACE FOR MAKING SHAPES

Got your phone? Great. Record this one and then play it back and incorporate this as part of your practice. If you do it a few mornings, you won't even need to play it; it will become part of your wake-up ritual.

This morning routine takes no more than ten minutes.

In the morning, while still in bed, place your hands on your heart, take three deep belly breaths—the exhale can be out your mouth or nose.

A deep belly breath is: like when you breathe through the nose and watch your belly inflate, (you are filling your lungs but are focused on your belly).

Now, remove your hands from the heart and rub them together— slowly at first, then create more friction and some heat.

Take that heat and warm your heart by pressing your warm hands downward, feeling the sensation of connecting with your heart space.

Next, tap firmly with two fingers—you can remove hands or just tap while hands are anchored. Hold an intention of awakening compassion as you tap. Do this for about a minute.

Stand, feel your feet press firmly on the ground. Reaching arms wide, look up, breathe deeply through the nose and sigh out the mouth, relaxing the face and squeezing shoulder blades together—make space in the front body. Do this for about a minute.

Ask yourself if you can identify with a feeling right now—sleepy, numb, out of it, kinda silly, curious, rushing, impatient.

Thank your heart for beating as you close your eyes and bring prayer hands to your heart. Then, repeat—aloud or internally—EhYah Asher EhYah.

EhYah Asher EhYah means I am that I am. It is an Old Testament name for God.

Remain connected to the ground. Stay present in your body, noting whatever you notice.

May your awakened heart remind you of gratitude for this ability to take a full breath, this delightful sip of chamomile tea, this old friend, this simple moment.

SPACE FOR MAKING SENSE

Your sacred space for making sense. You know what to do here.

WRiting Between the Chakras

And don't forget your stick-person and a 'heart chakra is here' mark on your body-doodle.

THE THROAT CHAKRA—THINK TRUTH

Located in the neck and the throat—including the thyroid which is a gland in the neck, essential for growth and maturation—this fifth chakra, color blue, element 'ether', reflects stress that is manifested in the inability or fear of speaking out.

When this chakra is overstimulated and out of balance, one might talk and gossip, resulting in drama. Do you know a person who never shuts up? I was one of those people. Never. Shut. Up. Oh, I'm sure sometimes people would want to tell me to, and maybe they did, but I wouldn't have heard them. I had too much unprocessed energy—unprocessed rage.

The foundation of imbalance in the throat chakra is trauma, verbal abuse, and excessive criticism. This can manifest in many problems with the ears, voice and neck. It can also show up as alcoholism and smoking/jewel addiction.

The demon of this chakra is lying.

To express a healthy throat chakra is to enhance communication. You can speak with authority and confidence—not heady and braggy—when expressing yourself.

One thing I did, early on, to contribute to healing my throat chakra, is take singing lessons. I felt Spirit call me to song to prepare for this book by addressing the judgment around my own voice.

Singing brings unity within as you utilize your breath and engage sound. I'm recalling biking nearby our home and singing to myself when suddenly a healing came up as I began shouting, "I can make noise! I can be loud! I can not sound pretty! I can sound ugly if I want to!"

An authentic voice is a perfect voice.

In my late thirties, I was singing in church—me, off key, boldly asking God: "If you give me a beautiful voice, I will use it to praise you."

As I began to write poetry, and record podcasts, people would say that they loved my voice. They'd say it was soothing. I took their loving words as a sign that I could continue to share my hard won wisdom. I also realized that God honored my prayer in a way I didn't anticipate.

I highly recommend chanting the seven Old Testament names for God, and have recorded them on the book's Youtube. Note: excess talking is a sign of unprocessed anger.

No one likes to be shushed. And I'm not suggesting we shush others or ourselves, but we can evaluate and modify where we are on the scale of gossip, untruths, dominating conversations, and simply too much talk and not enough action. Talk is cheap.

Subtlety comes in all those spaces between the words. Make more spaces than words. Try being the last to speak, taking in what everyone else has to say first. Ask yourself some questions that will help you move toward a healthier 'voice' and, ultimately, a balanced throat chakra.

Do you hate your voice when you hear yourself? Do you feel what you have to say is worth people listening or are you feeling the staleness of recycled conversation?

Record your voice on your phone and play it back. What came to mind? Perhaps, if you've recorded the movements in this book, you've already judged yourself.

Who is that inner critic? Hint: It's likely someone in your life from a long time ago, now a part of us in need of love.

Fear not, those voices are the people of the past... past relatives, past husbands... we hear them... we take them on as our own.

Explore what your own inner voice sounds like. Think what it would sound like if not influenced by those early critics. I am tempted to be prescriptive and suggest humming as a daily practice this week. Or maybe you already hum, whistle and sing all the day long?

A LETTER FOR YOU

Hey friends,

Paul here, the guy who never met Jesus while He walked the earth. So, in that way, I am just like you. I was chosen by God to be an apostle of our Messiah.

I'm writing this note to you, (reader fill in your name)_____, to tell you a bit about the truth and excellent news of your anointing.

May Abba himself infuse you with the fragrance of Christ's sweetness, the chrism; imparting total well-being. This aroma, like a gardenia, is electrifying as it re-charges every atom and fiber of your body. Those of you who embrace capital 'G' Grace will naturally extend love for the benefit of all. And, All means *all*. Those political affiliations must be diminished for Jesus' sake. Commit no longer to manufacture 'death' as in fearful thinking and speaking simply to prove yourself right. Political affiliations are a part of our temporal personalities. While conservatives may be focused on the glory days, progressives are equally guilty of rarely looking back and living in a dream-like future; the I AM is only ever right here in the present.

All of Abba's blessings from the heavenly realm have been lavished upon you, (your name)_____, as a loving gift from our sovereign Father —all because She sees you wrapped in Christ. Read that again—our Father who is in the heavenlies, *sees you*. It's personal. That is why we also call Him El Roi—the One who sees us. The One who sees is a nurturing mother. Can you see Him with Her mother/father face all bright smiles and warm chocolatey brown skin?

So you can celebrate this with all your heart! With all your soul! You were chosen, _____, yes *you!* to be Her very own, joining you to Himself even before He laid the foundation of the universe! She ordained you, so that you would be seen as holy in your Daddy's eyes.

After you fill in your name and re-read aloud to yourself, check in. How are you feeling about this intimacy and promise?

Chanting and the Chalice of Voice

I recognized I needed a breakthrough because all I could find inside was judgment and shame.

I realized I needed some compassion, to be gentler.

I closed my eyes, lying in my backyard hammock, and saw an image of a many–limbed, foreign, Hindu god. When I googled this image, I found out that the name was Avalokiteshvara.

He represents the mantra: Om Mani Padme Hum.

If I hadn't been doing yoga I wouldn't have received that image.

I began to chant it while walking the dog because it was said to carry the highest resonance of compassion.

And It worked... my heart began its healing and purification.

The thing is, if the voice is held in a chalice then it is not just holding chant, it's holding clarity.

A friend has said to me that she once saw me as so confused, but now I seem clear.

I explained that when I was confused, I didn't think I was confused.

What I didn't say was, now that I'm clear, I probably sound more confused than ever—to some. I've gone deeper. Clarity has taken me there.

Find your truth and speak it, sing it, write it, share it. With this writing, I am certain I am singing the song that I came onto the earth to sing. I was born with lots of pure songs in my heart. You were too— may you allow them to be birthed from your tongue.

Living in the truth of our identity is the freedom of feeling clear, not clogged by the memory of trauma. Once the old yeast has been spread around to balance chakra energies pertaining to inherited ignorance and blind spots, the newly released prana points us to the choices we have to help confront issues: e.g. large systemic, societal issues of inequality and racism.

The revelation of God's true power in the Bible is from the perspective of the oppressed. The gospel reveals a liberating path of humility, compassion, and nonviolence in the face of evil.

So what happened?

Father Rohr summarizes simply:

"For the first three hundred years after Jesus' death, Christians were the oppressed minority. But by the year 400 C.E., Christians had changed places. We moved from hiding in the catacombs to presiding in the basilicas. That is when we started reading the Bible, not as subversive literature,

the story of the oppressed, but as establishment literature to justify the status quo of people in power. When Christians began to gain positions of power and privilege, they began to ignore... the Sermon on the Mount."

But when we invite the East, it introduces us to an open, transformed mind; one in which we realize we have been battling with our physical bodies out of fear of illness and death because the culture puts them in an egoic light, to be viewed through a worldly lens. Our bodies need liberation from the tyranny of a fear-based mindset. Pure undifferentiated Christ consciousness sits beneath and undergirds the rational mind.

The goal is for body and soul to no longer be at odds. Let's venture out of the box. Let's toss that box; we won't be needing it.

Write this, then read aloud:

Dear body:

Relax. I'm laying down my word weapons—the hurtful stories I tell myself—at your feet.

I come in peace.

You, oh body, are a vessel of truth in a temple of divine consciousness.

SPACE FOR MAKING SHAPES

Record it on your phone, bathe in your own words as you play it back and participate in the practice. Come lie on your belly for cobra and sphinx poses. For cobra I invite you to come onto finger tips with your elbows bent and wide to the sides of your mat. Press down into your hips and lower body, firm your belly before lifting your face and shoulders on an inhale. Look right, then left...again. Exhale lower your forehead down. pause breathe in and out. Then repeat 3-5 more cobras.

For sphinx you will bring your elbows down and closer to your ribs with your hands now palms flat. Inhale press into forearms and life face, shoulders wide, feeling breath fill your heart. Stay for 8-10 breaths, pressing firmly with your lower body grounded.

There are many ways to build resilience in life, but using our physical bodies to enter and stay in discomfort is one simple and powerful way. Take chair pose for example:

Stand to Bring your knees and feet just a few inches apart and drop your seat with your weight now more in your heels. Feel the strength of your own quads as you reach your arms up by your ears. Breathe in, breathe out. Stay.

You are taking your seat of righteousness. Stay. Witness discomfort.

Stay

because you can.

Stay because as you focus on the power of your legs and your breath

you are building an interior focused on this Zoe life. This life which brings peace and power into the world. God's loving, healing power to liberate us all from the chains of oppression. Come in and out of your chair posture 5-10 more times. Just be present.

Now—

Take figure 4 to open the hips. You can do this seated or lying on your back. Cross right ankle onto left knee. Draw your chest and your figure 4 closer to feel sensation. Breathe imagining you are creating space in the tight hip. My husband lets out loud exhales and groans when I help him stretch his tight hips. Switch sides. Notice what came to mind. We yoga teachers are known to quip, "Let your mother out of your hip."

Rest in corpse pose for 5-10 minutes

Be sure that your muscles will remind you of this work tomorrow. Be sure and thank them!

SPACE FOR MAKING SENSE

Here you go again. In a magnificent expression of you. Whether you
question, define, list words you want to look up, create your own
quote. Do some or all as a statement from your heart.

Writing Between the Chakras

And, do your map of Self with a sketch of you. Perhaps this time you'll
be in a thought bubble, or you'll have mastered the stick person sitting
cross-legged. No matter the position, mark the throat chakra.

THE THIRD EYE CHAKRA—THINK KNOWER

The light of the body is the eye: if therefore thine eye be single,
thy whole body shall be full of light.

MATTHEW 6:22

Located between the brows, this chakra is about perceiving. Holy Spirit opened my eyes. I see beyond my mask. I see beyond yours as well.

The third eye is the eye of the heart. Its color is Indigo. All about intuition, the third eye sees through the lens of love, truth, and non-duality. To walk like Jesus—in Truth + Love, is to walk with God.

I'm no expert in neuroscience, but it would be beneficial to read about the happenings in the pineal and pituitary glands and their activation of spiritual revelations and optimal health.

Is it any surprise that the sixth chakra's element is light? If the eyes are the window to the soul, then what does that third eye open up to, view, and reflect?

My cousin, more than 20 years my junior, told me a few years back that she had a vision of me. There I stood with a big bunch of colorful flowers growing from the top of my head. But then the blossoms closed up and she heard: 'she'll need to go through the fire before they are restored.'

You know what my knee jerk response was? Fuck that. Fuck that vision. Why? Because, at that point, I had been through a decade of entering and sitting in the fire. I was tired. And feeling a little too crispy.

Yet this chakra of *light* requires more fire to keep burning up all the ignorance we carry. There is no substitute for knowing truth— the truth about who we are. Self-esteem based on achievement is acquired. It's contingent, fickle. True self-esteem is birthed from our doing nothing the world would call deserving of esteem. It's a graced gift everyone was given simply by being born.

And on that day with my cousin, I did not yet embody love from the tip of my toes to the top of my head. The reason? I still carried a deep, dark secret which had been festering, making me fiery in all the 'wrong' places—I still wasn't aligned with my truth.

In a hands-down easy opposite, the third eye's demon is illusion. Like a head in the sand, close the eyes and imagine what you want to see, rather than what is truly there. The Spirit gives clear insight to things as they are- before we can label, divide and judge.

You can tap that spot right now. It is responsible for the connection between Spirit and the outer world. When it is in balance, you can see both the inner and outer worlds from singleness. A healthy third eye or brow chakra allows you clear thought and self-reflection; connected to God's Spirit vs. ego-based fear. You can build it like a muscle, this intuitive knowing.

An example is how I created this book with 'someone else'. Part of the learning means practicing a less analytical, less rational approach, and understanding that there is much that is out of our direct control.

Motivated by knowledge—reflected, learned, and intuitive—this chakra represents your connection to wisdom and insight. It lets you access an inner guidance system from deep within. You can, when it's in balance, cut through what's temporal (the illusion) and access deeper truth.

Mindfulness is associated with the sixth chakra. It helps you live in the present moment. The third eye chakra is connected to logic and to creativity—strength in each allows you to be innovative. A Christian student recently commented to me that yoga and breathing practice have helped her tap into healing and surrender. She sees that a 'thinker' like herself, a traditional woman of the faith, has wisdom available to her through her body. She says she is in awe of what she's learning.

In my own life, my intuition had been invalidated. I was denied the true identity of my birth father for thirty-eight years. This did not start with me either. Yes, a pattern.

There are often, in social media, stories—short videos—of 'father in the service has been away and surprises the child'. These vignettes have been shared for decades—ever the heartwarming reunion of a military man and his family; always pulling at the heartstrings of the viewer.

Suddenly, in my mid-forties, I found myself bursting into tears watching one of those videos.

You see, the man in my mother's wedding picture, the man I thought was my father, was dressed in a navy uniform. My little girl inside, never having met him, desperately wanted one of those stories to happen to me. I realized, in that moment, how many times I, as a little girl, I must have longed for daddy to surprise me at school or

at least on my birthday. I ended up despising birthday celebrations.
Every picture revealed a scowl. Funny, for most of my life I mistakenly
thought I was just a spoiled brat. How wrong. And how sorry. Oh,
little Anita I see you, I feel you.

I don't have many memories of my childhood (a common symptom
of CPTSD which I only learned about in recent years) but I imagine
every year at Christmas I must have decided to stuff down the desire
for my father's return—complete with a big bag of presents for his
only child. Eventually, I just stopped asking.

When we've created the subconscious wishes, and are called to
heal these 'false stories that are connected to our identity', we face
challenges.

At those times, know this: your intuition can serve you well.

"Your intuition is yours for you to develop
and it is to be used in service to humanity."

TOMMY ROSEN, INTERNATIONALLY RENOWNED YOGA TEACHER
AND CREATOR OF RECOVERY 2.0 LIFE BEYOND ADDICTION

For years, the stories I was being told didn't go with what I felt in
my heart was true. I kept looking at that wedding photo. There was
always something off. This shut down the intuitive aspect of me for
decades. Remember, I wasn't always where I am now. I was without a
diagnosis, ashamed, alone, angry and scared.

I learned not to trust myself.

In your life, have you had to grieve for what you thought your life was
going to look like?

We have a higher vision. It sees beyond what the open eyes can see. It goes deeper than the physical eyes process. It's a gift to see with the single eye, from the heart's depths. Some days, especially during the Covid pandemic, my energy body became so filled with the anxiety of our world that I found myself taking meditative, eyes-closed pauses, almost every hour. It manifests as profoundly feeling the shift into anxiety as I am no longer calm and present while reading online. I am suddenly plunged into a sense of rushing or lostness. Fortunately, because of a decade of practices, I know how to find the peace within and rather quickly. Within our moment of pause we might recall: anxiety is harbored survival energy .I am actually ok.

But I first learned of that pause nearly eight years ago while in the park with my dog during the winter when the ground was covered in three feet of snow. I had been waking each day for weeks with anxiety in my chest and had no idea what it was from or how to address it. On this day, in the park, I decided to ask God to help me. That's when I heard clearly to lie down.

"Now?" I asked. "In the snow?"

There was no response.

See, it's up to me to move, to do the action. As soon as I lay my body on the earth, the anxiety seeped out of me. This was the beginning of my embodied understanding of nature bringing the nervous system into coherence. I began to see my nervous system having dissociated for so long as heroic. I began to see this as an example of restoring the Mother, the feminine, the yin.

Paracelsus, the 16th-century German-Swiss physician, gave voice to that same intuition when he wrote, *"The art of healing comes from nature, not from the physician."*

Then there is the Eastern proverb *"Shin to bul ee."* Body and soil are one.

Sounds like from dust we came and dust we shall return.

I've noticed more people, those who maybe formerly didn't have time to spend outdoors, now spend time in nature during their quarantine/shelter in place. Maybe you've felt especially cooped up and claustrophobic?

That got me thinking about the multitude of times during my life I ached to be free of a situation, feeling powerless. I was stuck in a job I despised for over a decade. My husband and I were stuck, suffering unexplained infertility for over three years. There were probably thousands of times, while in stuck, I despised my Self. Stuck because of sin cycles that would not break. Looking back I did not know I had choices. Patterns of existence seemed ingrained.

Are you feeling stuck and powerless right now? In what ways? Write it down here, or take it to the 'Space For Making Sense' section.

Then write to your future Self. For example: I see you in your new job feeling creative and grateful.

Do your stretching and shaking practices. What is lodged in the mind will be moved gently by the body. A new path will be revealed. Trust your God has your back.

How Do We Know the Third Eye Is There?

What comes to mind are some friends who are blind. It is clear that, when one part of our typical way of operating is taken away, another aspect of our senses is developed. The blind operate with other senses. It is truly amazing to witness their walk in faith, all their other senses heightened.

To use the third eye, accessing all the chakras, feeling the inner child being in Him, is to walk in faith. At that point we've surrendered our beliefs that we once relied upon. We take a huge risk when we already feel somewhat enlightened, so why push the envelope to feel further discomfort? Why put myself there? Why put yourself there? For God's promises, and to adhere to His call. He is a bottomless well of love and of moral revival. The fear of surrendering for our own sanctification is the pattern of dying and rising, and can be trusted when our nervous systems are in equanimity. If you're afraid of Good Friday, you'll never experience Resurrection Sunday.

When it comes to surrender and opening, there are two options as I see it: 1) we are present and coming from the compassionate, open heart which experiences suffering, and we embrace it because we're a part of the beauty and love of that embrace. Or 2) we are asleep. We're in fear. We're numb. The tomb is still blocked by that stone.

But we follow a God who's in the rolling stone business.

Before I saw with my single eye, I spent so much time in my head in the past and in the future. I was never in the present learning to trust the energy of the body—therefore, I was never really fully alive in the moment.

The unobserved Self, that didn't have faith, was in survival, behaving in a primal way. Urges and popularity. The urges ran me. They run us. This is normal and human, and all included in our journey to wholeness. These lower energies must come under the power of the mind of Christ, which is a natural outflowing of East meeting West. Our physical brains are the basis of renewing our minds. (Similar ideas are expressed in Rom 12:2). When we operate from our triune brain: head, heart, and gut, we enjoy thoughts from an endless source of inspiration. Our imaginations light up and we are continually amazed with this sense of freedom.

After those urges run us, we feel shame. For example: oh, I ate that whole cake, again. Oh, I told that same lie, again. What if we flip those lines to: naturally I make lots of mistakes in my hu-maning journey.

I am quite certain these invitations to showing up fully are like calls to the carpet asking us to surrender to what is larger than the small self. These calls encourage us to do all we can so that we develop a new way to see.

Doing the 'work' of uniting the inner child to your divine Self may be difficult, but not doing it is downright irresponsible. It challenges us to have our West open the door to East. Eventually you will never step back through the door toward bondage and delusion. The work doesn't have to feel heavy. The Father was good before the incarnation of the Son. The Father has always been united to His Sons of humanity and His love is unmatched.

Awareness can be painful, like a too bright sun causing a burn. But, oh, divine is the taste of peace that follows. Think: the future you thanking the you of today for your efforts. Think: you stopping to try to be a 'better person' thus fully embodying the imperfect you that you already are. It's a paradox— sure I'm a little broken, but I am also so whole.

Be brave, dear reader. Become like the athlete who brings everything out onto the field and leaves it all there. Keep going.

What am I asking you to do? Participate in a divine exchange. Hand something to God: your fears and stories. Trust that God will offer back gifts for sharing. But mostly trust this budding relationship with the Son. Trust that through those gifts you will meet the brave and bold you—the one that is partially hidden. The one made ready to participate in the life of being God's family. You have the divine nature!

When you bring everything out to the field, you will discover your team/tribe—you have never been alone. Being a kamikaze yogi is not a path of transcending the ordinary, but fully realizing the beauty in it. It is not a path of rising above the rest of humanity, but of becoming truly grounded in humble truth.

What I'm learning about Christ, and the seven chakras, and the seven churches, and the hu-man I am with deep roots, with instinct, is that this is a power I can handle when I am in collaboration with God, and when I am in service to the community.

At these times—which is mostly always—I'm filled, then propelled, by a supernatural power that I realize the world may not be able to understand. And that's okay. It's okay that not everyone or anyone understands my transfiguration. I don't always get it. But when I feel I am the church, I am the poured out wine, the broken bread, I know that my heart is open, as is my vision. The reason we know the world won't understand can be found in Matthew 7:13 The Passion Translation:

"The Narrow Gate—Come to God through the narrow gate, because the wide gate and broad path is the way that leads to destruction—nearly everyone chooses that crowded road! The narrow gate and the difficult way leads to eternal life—so few even find it!"

Wildly and wonderfully, enlightenment is as close as your hand on your heart, and it feels like the eucharist walking around in the world. Living this way is freedom sourced in confidence. And it allows each enlightened one to remain in their own lane, doing what they are charged to do-gazing straight without that constant looking left then right.

It's like that for me. In my own lane—swimming under that infinity sign—confident in my mission. Arguments fall away, the news of the world does not rattle me. Even I am surprised to hear myself proclaim that there is a king who reigns, and so no earthly leader is made to compete.

My hope is that every human knows they are the beloved and the verse to summarize it best is John 14:20 "In that day, Jesus says, you will know that I am in my Father and you are in me and I am in you"

That, in building a relationship with East, and knowing a Jesus that embraces all, you can boldly bring the world unique gifts formed from your release of control.

You'll stop doubting if you did enough because you loved well.

The Bible speaks of transforming the mind, the kingdom of heaven is now and within. Try saying aloud—we are in heaven now, a dimension of God's creation.

That's what the transformation means. It is the genesis of your life. When that happens, it is the beginning of discovering the truth of your identity. Maybe the mystics of today are those that have been traumatized by life's stresses and abuses. The body became unsafe to occupy in the present so we learned to dissociate as a survival mechanism.

The long journey back into the body creates a safe haven for the Spirit of God to dwell. I am dramatically lost and just as dramatically found.

The gospel good news is especially powerful for the individual who has experienced the most pain in this lifetime. These people are the wounded who have now become healers. We include ourselves in this modern-day Sermon on the Mount. To be lowly like Mother Mary is a posture of humility and openness. To be virginal is to be self-possessed.

From theologian N.T. Wright: " ... *the method of the kingdom will match the message of the kingdom. The kingdom will come as the church, energized by the Spirit, goes out into the world vulnerable, suffering, praising, praying, misunderstood, misjudged, vindicated, celebrating: always—as Paul puts it in one of his letters—bearing in the body the dying of Jesus so that the life of Jesus may also be displayed.*"

This puts us in the posture of a vulnerable servant of the suffering world. We are called to participate and be challenged to keep looking at the messes, including ourselves as part of the problem, and so empowered now to be part of the solution. We won't feel safe to be misunderstood and judged if our body's own nervous system shuts down due to chronic stress.

I'm a big fan of podcasts. On a recent episode of *Another Name for Everything*, James Finlay's work was featured as a modern contemplative. This is an Eastern attribute. To contemplate. To imagine, ponder, wonder. That's a big part of what we do when we journey within, and when we take these steps of trust.

"The contemplative way is like a monastery without walls, a gathering place for people who are searching for something more—something more meaningful, intimate, and richly present to the gift of their own life."

JAMES FINLAY

I went a long time needing to find that 'something more'. Right in the midst of mothering, being a wife and nanny and then yoga teacher. Then I found it, my monastery without walls. Christ our mother fills the human unmet need for those who were, as infants and children, separated from parental love. There are many commonplace childhood wounds that are not traumatizing. For example, a critical parent, or feeling left out, or experiencing the pain of being misunderstood. And there are childhood traumas which can cause C-PTSD: low to no attunement, neglect, abandonment and abuse. All are cause for our inner child to turn to Him for connection and rest in the everlasting arms.

For a season, as I learned about the inner life of me, in Christ, I felt misunderstood and odd. But then, true to the cycles of faith, He brought me back into the world with new awareness. So at times it feels like this: I'm in the interior, dark womb space, safe and secure, familiar now with the terrain. Then when it is time to re-engage with the world, I say to Him, "I need to know you are in all of this life with me! I'm afraid I won't sense your nearness like I do when we are quiet together."

But I am assured somehow to be bold and confident that indeed my Jesus is Lord overall. We aren't to hide our wisdom under a bushel. Every day the same damn message, which I have inked on my left forearm: Talitha koumi.

Yes, those words 'Talitha koumi' are so direct and healing. Arise, little one. Two words which allow the rich to see their disconnection from the perceived poor, and from which the poor might find empowerment, energy, and tools for change and healing.

Arise, little one. And that, my friends, often feels terrifying.

It is true. We never need to be hungry for parental love again. We can become unafraid. We can begin by valuing the lost parts of ourselves.

I like to think of Jesus, Son of Man, entering time and space in a particular way, but we are charged with discovering all that is timeless and spaceless about Him and know these aspects of Self: mind, body + spirit not one superior to the others.

STAND ALONE

God Sees You (El Roi)

Whenever we create without God, when we force, when we scheme for selfish, greedy purposes, we are seen. Our own soul sees us. I imagine she shrinks.

In Genesis, Sarah, wife of Abraham, assigned Hagar—her servant girl—to be a surrogate. This is how Ishmael (he plays a foundational role in Islamic tradition) was born. Sarah then became cruel to Hagar—derived from her envy over Hagar's fertility. So she evicted Hagar and her new baby (Abraham's son).

Hagar and her infant were left to their own devices in the wilderness, alone and afraid. In her desperation, she cried out to God. He answered.

Hagar, this powerless, Egyptian slave answered God by name, praying to the God who spoke to her and calling Him El Roi. She acknowledged it by saying that he was the God who saw her.

> *"Yes! He saw me; and then I saw him!" Gen 16:13*
>
> MESSAGE TRANSLATION

When we use other humans for our pleasure and personal gain we are not of a clear, loving heart.

But Christ is not one to punish, but redeem. What we thought was done while we were yet sinning is *always* purposed by God for reconciliation, for the world's benefit.

Jesus will never objectify us. His penetration—the Light of truth, is always to bring freedom, and foster a deeper relationship. I've been known to quip that Jesus threw the first stone. If you have not begun the deconstruction of your false Self, you will hear this with confused ears. Yet, Isaiah 32 assures us "Each man will be like a shelter from the wind and a refuge from the storm.... the eyes of those who see will no longer be closed."

We are Hagar whenever we feel scared, alone, demoralized, and helpless in the wilderness of our life: abandoned to the elements, uncertain of our future, desperate to have our basic needs met. I do believe this is how my own mother must have felt when my birth father left us immediately after I was born, repeating the pattern of abandonment from the past he was handed.

Hagar is every Woman (every human)
our shadow sexuality
the hidden slave girl
not the proper face we show the world
not queenly and put together
nor pedigreed
but the body unattached from
a noble head
a body purposed
a body exposed
a body procreation-focused to move humanity forward
single use

discarded
objectified
fugitive
illegitimate
utilitarian

There is something we can all do to ease all of the previous burdens.

Yoga is one practice which purposes a yoking of mind and body, revealing the hurting, enslaved you to your true Self dancing within a glorious trinity.

How might you be numbing or hiding this part of you?

The gospel of dependency on God can make sense at ever deeper levels. If you, like me, are a white, middle-class woman who does not typically identify as scorned or rejected, it doesn't take much to connect to our ancestors or other women around the world who live this way. It's the essence or spirit of Hagar in each human who has this authority—once we identify how we feel persecuted, worthless, abused, or oppressed.

She is a model of strength through her self-liberating drive. Every ripple of healing which trembles through your body sends forth a call to the Mother for a tsunami of grace to greet the shores of our suffering world. For certainly God will move when we do.

SPACE FOR MAKING SHAPES

Lie down on your back for happy baby.
Grab for your knees and draw them wide to stretch your groin.
Find your breath slowing now and deepening.
Either leave your hands on your knees and relax your shoulders and
jaw or grab your feet if they are accessible.

This taking of another 'baby shape'
communicates at a deep level to your inner child. Just be present in
your body and notice your thoughts, maybe your memories?

After three or four minutes, come to lie curled up on your side in
fetal position. Feel close to yourself and bring to mind your face as
an infant. Say to that infant Self: "I've got you. You are safe with me".

Next—

Make a fist and then cover the right fist with left hand; hold tightly

God wanted you here
you're covered and protected
you're connected
you are truly one
there's no separation
you couldn't pull the hand away if you tried.
switch it—cover your left fist now
Jesus is the infant fist and you're in charge of protecting him
this new life growing in you, precious cargo to remember
we realize that this is the challenge of self-abandonment

how many times we left ourselves exposed, maybe even in danger
we didn't know better
we didn't know that we were put in charge of this little life.
This death energy overtakes us and we're foolish
and we don't care for the Self
it's like a death wish isn't it?
We don't understand our worthiness
we don't understand what we're here to do
we don't understand the power we've been given
and you can't pinpoint it—because it's in our cervix and in our feet
it's in our heart and in our brain, and that's why we have to learn to
bring a curiosity and ultimately a sacred attitude toward our bodily
functions, our limitations and, most especially our lovemaking

SPACE FOR MAKING SENSE

You know what to do with this. Write, journal, jot down questions.

Writing Between the Chakras

Can you doodle yourself again, and place the chakras you've become aware of. What is the setting like around you? How is that illustrated? Where does the energy stop? Does it?

THE CROWN CHAKRA—THINK UNITY

I feed my crown chakra a purple smoothie first thing in the morning: blueberries, spinach, beets, and banana, blended into a violet hue.

Picture me, a woman of 54, riding my bike around my neighborhood singing a little tune when, suddenly, the Knower shows me a way to best describe my mind prior to integrating the energy of my body and how it feels now. I stopped my bike and spoke into my phone recorder.

Pre-kingdom mind was like an 8-lane highway, busy with traffic, jam-packed with other vehicles. All that exhaust, all that honking. Can you see it? So many drivers trying to get somewhere. In. my. mind.

Kingdom mind is just me in my car on the same 8-lane highway with all that lovely space in all directions. All that quiet. Just nature surrounding me and I get to play whatever I want on the radio with no distractions. Or I can just be. Enjoying the ride.-

The seventh chakra is often depicted as a lotus flower atop the head, and symbolically described as having one thousand petals. Crown is violet, and associated with bright, golden light—as in pure light. Its element is thought.

The crown chakra is cosmic consciousness—something we each carry. Through this divine seat of awareness we are connected to the eternal (remember eternal includes now—it is not some future time). It sounds so ethereal and, without a balanced root, it is. Some people are overly spiritualized. They cannot seem to connect to the present reality. Maybe they wish to bypass being in a messy body, thereby projecting their disgust onto other messy bodies.

Though many might mark the chakras on the body, as they appear on popular posters, the crown chakra is infinite; it begins at the crown of the head and continues off into the ether.

When our crown chakra is balanced, we feel connected to our higher Self—meaning our best Self and most informed, wise, and peaceful Self. This Self is not God, but be assured: She is made in the image of God. When Jesus looks in the mirror who do you think He sees? She is imperfect and feels fine about that. She is both broken and whole and understands there is always a third way being birthed from the willingness to embrace paradox.

We are sourced in an ocean of serenity. May this book be a 'how to' manual to open and reveal the truth you long to experience firsthand. Venture to shift belief into knowing the divine as He is expressed in the world in and through you. There is a fancy theological term for this mutual indwelling without loss of personhood: perichoresis.

When the chakra is imbalanced or blocked, we can suffer from depression, a sense of alienation even. It is difficult for us to feel empathy for others when our crown chakra is not in balance. Disruption in the crown tends to come from living in stressful environments, and is linked to fast-paced lifestyles. God cannot join us in our busy-ness. Unresolved trauma that is deeply rooted and aligns negatively with our core beliefs (developed in childhood) blocks the crown chakra.

When we think the same conditioned thoughts as our parents, we know we are not in creation mode. When we are habitually scrolling and consuming on social media, again, not creating. Simply put, we are either creating or destroying and the best place to initiate imagination is from the serenity of a quiet body-mind. Both alert and relaxed.

Say aloud: I was made to create.

An imbalanced energy center impacting the hippocampus and amygdala develops into hidden chronic stress, increasing cortisol throughout the entire system, and can include:

Apathy/depression
Lack of care and compassion towards others
Excessive bragging
Insomnia
Nightmares/night terror
Boredom
Feeling of alienation from others
Narrow-mindedness/dogmatism
Spiritual disconnection
Rigid and limiting self-identity
Greed and materialism
Mental fog/confusion
Loneliness
Physical inflammation.

Before my crown opened, I used to think ugly thoughts: recycled stuff from the day before; a conveyor belt of sad and murky thoughts. I'd dive into fantasy—imaginings which demonstrated dissatisfaction with where I was in my ordinary life.

I'm reminded of tears in warrior pose during a public class in downtown Philly recently. The teacher's theme was mental health. My body responded in a profound way because I had no idea that I had recovered from a form of mental illness. I thought my struggles were normal—I'd minimized them my entire life, even journaling about being 'satisfied with my body and my Spirit, but my brain would probably always be a little broken'. I had no idea I could experience such a beautiful and renewed mind.

Most people's thoughts are about eighty percent repetitive of what they were thinking the day before. Seriously. Sad, isn't it? But then think of the potential. Whatever number you estimate for yourself, the challenge is to meet yourself, again and again, with compassion and awareness.

You may find yourself wondering what is wrong with you .There's nothing wrong with you—just keep doing your practices. Move that energy.

Jesus gifts me a vision: He and I conjoined twins connected at the crown... curled up.

Bringing the crown chakra into balance requires self-awareness at the highest level. One of the most effective ways of balancing is medita- tion. Meditation allows one to discover the true Self. I was not ready for silent, still meditation until I had prepared my body for years with breath-led movements on my yoga mat releasing decades of pent up 'story' about my chronic pain. That is why there are a total of eight limbs to yoga and the asana or shapes are just one. Yoga, in all its rich, ancient history and tradition includes paths of devotion, study, philosophy, and service.

The feelings we experience and the 'cellular level changes' that occur as a result of gratitude are astounding. The more you give thanks, the more you speak of envisioning a loving world, the more you serve to build that world—using your own inspired thinking.

Yoga leads to God, or it is nothing.

FR. JEAN-MARIE DÉCHANET, AUTHOR: CHRISTIAN YOGA

More on the Crown Chakra

In the Christian tradition, the Crown chakra would be the mind of Christ—the blueprint of the logic for the meaning behind the *new breed* of human: humans who live in a world of each caring for the other. Because we know, but for the grace of God, go I. Politics aside, we must do better for the least of these.

The crown connects us to universal aspects that are beyond the Self. We are transported, through the power of this energy center, from I to I am, from me to we—a unifying of the mind, left and right brain operating as one. Head, heart, and gut, a single operating system. The corpus callosum sends signals back and forth without a veil to separate and divide. Righteousness or the Hebrew, tsedeq, will restore quietness, securing a place within—undisturbed, blessed. Only the fool in us practices ungodliness, often resulting in devastating consequences for the powerless. We want to share our power if we have any at all.

I have experienced unitive consciousness (higher than mundane, higher than ordinary existence) like people do on psilocybin, simply because my brain, like all brains, can be altered by meditation and the power of my own breath. Brain chemicals can flood us with a 'high', and these moments will change us. Because, in this state, the default mode network is quieted. From here the ego becomes less and less fearful that she is separate from God. After a certain point, she never questions her placement in Him.

I spent years inside my abandonment wound thinking it was unique to me because of my actual abandonment by my birth father. But it turns out many people operate from a core fear of being left alone even if this didn't happen while still young. We can arrive at a 'found' aspect of our embodied Soul so that we never have to worry about feeling alone again. Jesus is truly our forever companion. Goodbye boredom, goodbye loneliness.

In his latest book, *How to Change Your Mind*, Michael Pollan writes of his own consciousness-expanding experiments with psychedelic drugs like LSD and psilocybin, and he makes the case for why shaking up the brain's old habits could be therapeutic for people facing addiction and depression.

We become liberated from small-mindedness. Our vision for human-ity expands from personal experience. We find we are praying for enemies, not because a priest told us to, but because there is a person praying through us now, and the prayer flowing through us is for everyone to discover it is a Christ-soaked world: mercy restored.

Connected at the crown, you and Christ, me and Christ, we bloom a new petal in the lotus of the crown. When I can successfully get out of my own way, I can tell God's love story for humanity through my own brave journey of battling demons. It's a story like Jesus' where I find myself victor.

Would you pause right here and put on 'Landslide' by Fleetwood Mac? Try belting it out, dancing around and allowing these lyrics to penetrate your heart: *"Oh, mirror in the sky, what is love? Can the child within my heart rise above."*

You are almost done reading this book and I am inviting you into one final participaction with the concept of 'as above so below'. You, feeling the love pouring down from above, while pouring out from your center.

Let us return to the mystic Julian of Norwich as she observes, *"If I pay special attention to myself, I am nothing at all; but in general, I am, I hope, in the unity of love… for it is in this one-ing that the life of all people consists…"*

She reflects: *"The love of God creates in us such a one-ing that, when it is truly seen, no person can separate themselves from another."*

Finally, let us hear Julian, in her own Middle English words, speaking of divine and human unity: *"For in the sighte of God alle man is one man, and one man is alle man."*

One life, one death, one Spirit.

It's been this way for thousands of years right here in our tradition and yet most did not have the wholeness of mind to conceive the truth as Jesus revealed. Our nervous system regulating will allow us to become more comfortable living the pattern of death and rebirth, repentance, and resurrection. We dive deeper to grow in our tradition, and we watch as love and wisdom bloom.

One of my favorite maxims is 'how is life happening for me?' I had to look deeply at how and why I was sabotaging my beautiful life (hint: death energy). Why did I seem unable to fully enjoy the gifts I was given? I was angry at my chronic IBS, my poorly functioning brain. I was sabotaging my own growth and finally, I was unable to handle my embarrassing emotional swings (sign of a wounded inner child).

What do you sabotage?
What are you angry at or about?
Do you know why?

> *"This resurrection life you received from God is not a timid, grave-tending life. It's adventurously expectant, greeting God with a childlike 'What's next, Papa?'"*
>
> ROM 8:15 MSG

If sin is dead, when we sin we are reacting from a now identified place of death within. This moment or state or season of brokenness is the pivot we make toward relationship. As mentioned, I am finishing this book during COVID-19 as the summer of Black Lives Matter marches heat up after the murder of George Floyd. I do believe Mr. Floyd's unspeakably violent and haunting death is the hinge upon which our new reality opens.

Thousands have taken to the streets in protest and many are violently expressing rage. Most are not, most are peaceful. And yet, the voices of the Old Testament prophets have warned us that, if we do not listen to the cries of the oppressed, do not be surprised when their righteous anger blows up as holy rage. If we have created and sustained an unjust system, there will be a necessary deconstruction before the rebuilding. There will be a necessary season of repentance and deep lament before revival.

If you yourself have never given expression to the wildness of your pain, you probably fear this intensely. I get it. The heart understands the paradox. Is it ugly? Of course. Is it necessary? Of course. Like a storm clears the building tensions of humidity.

It occurs when we forget who we are. One could say every person has the occasional amnesia of identity in the mind. Never in the body, however. The body cannot lie.

For seven years, now with discipline, and seven before, with casual curiosity, I have committed to getting on my mat daily to explore what these words mean: Ez 36:7 *"…and I will lay sinews upon you, and will cause flesh to come upon you, and cover you with skin, and put breath in you, and you shall live, and you shall know that I am the LORD— to know I am offspring of the Divine."*

I would pay attention to where I was in a state of fear, lust, lying, illusion, and ask Him to show me ultimate reality. How can I see this—even be this—and your Word says something different? How am I who you say I am? Must I travel through my limbic system evolutionary-style as if I were becoming homo-erectus. Must I know my animal natures one by one? Must I abhor my inability to control my emotions and my thoughts? Is a man just pretending to be upright and moral if he does not visit his lower nature and explore what is true ultimately? If man lives in subconscious fear of what he's capable of, can he ever truly be certain he won't break and commit an unforgivable sin?

I do not recall how it dawned on me that what I was experiencing in my body—the repeated cycles of letting go, crying out, facing shame—would then point me to my bible, a book I had resisted reading. A book I knew nothing about. Isn't that a miracle? A living God who would show me the ancient words as confirmation of my own rebirth as a woman made of His spirit. A brave, resilient woman who stopped being afraid of what I was being shown about myself. The great divide would be obvious and there was no leap to a better me. I would have to keep loving and having the highest compassion for me just as I was.

But this Jesus of mine would never leave me there. Somehow, I would find myself gently moved beyond my former ways. We were brilliantly designed 'not to be fixed'. We are not a problem to fix. I am not a problem to fix. You are not a problem to fix. And yet the ways we operate can cause dis-ease. Patterns in relationships may create upset and hopelessness. For this is where we say we feel stuck. Stuck is a place from where we can become unstuck. Let's just name that. We'll start by being on our knees every day. When we submit that way, the power available to us is infinite and unfathomable. Say "Kneeling is my superpower" smiling all the while.

> *"For we have the living Words full of energy and it pierces*
> *more sharply than a double-edged sword. It will penetrate to the*
> *very core of our being where soul and spirit, bone and marrow joint meet.*
> *It interprets and reveals true thoughts, the secret motives*
> *of our hearts."*
>
> HEB 4:12 PASSION TRANSLATION

Religiosity lied to us about Abba's goodness. If we cannot trust our Father then we will hide, deny and blame-shift our missteps. If you never try, you'll never know your true worth.

If I'm always trying to control myself—be on my best behavior—then that is not being true to the death of Christ in me that I, like every human, carry within. I recognize there's healing—something dormant in me, now resurrected. True intimacy with Christ is discovered in the dark, in the shadows and in our great need. Any of our human tendencies to destroy (gossip, lying, greed, violence to Self or other in thought word or deed) stunts flourishing and therefore points us toward the underlying sickness simply manifesting as the symptoms of sin and ignorance.

There's a purpose to misstep. Error, reflection on how wrong we continue to be, gets us closer to the truth because, if we don't get beyond good behavior we don't grow.

Is sin a manifestation of pain and discord inside us? Many psychologists are telling us right now that the roots of white supremacy, having to be in power, is found in our inner child landscape of disconnection from our caregivers. A signal that a deeper wound is in need of healing. Insistence on always being good is fatal because it will put a cap on your growth and your holiness which is derived from repentance. Remember, objectively you are already whole and holy, but subjectively we work all of this out in our broken relationships and by letting go of our compulsive need to be seen as good. We are learning to trust God to see our 'bad'.

What do you think?

Christ has been in us all along, but veiled by the indoctrinated type of thinking we've absorbed from various lessons and churches. In short, too much Westness and not enough Eastness.

"Faith is about realizing Jesus Christ in you, in the midst of contradiction! Just as ore is placed into a crucible, where the dross is separated

from the gold in a furnace, come to the conclusion for yourselves
of his indwelling! Should it appear to you that Christ is absent in
your life, look again, you have obviously done the test wrong!"

2 COR 13:5 MIRROR BIBLE

There was a time when I almost left my husband. I ranted, screamed, and worse—completely in blame mode. I packed a bag, went to the car, and drove away. But I didn't even end my rant there. I drove back and kept that negative engine rolling, stepping back into the house and making accusations. I said I would sleep in the car. I made a massive event—the whole time I was sinning, out of control for six hours.

The wise and peaceful warrior of a husband knew that this was stagnant energy I was dealing with. He remained calm and refused to engage, so the energy kept dying—despite my reviving it over and over and over.

He took an enormous risk, this warrior—oftentimes worrier—husband of mine. Bob trusted God's plan; he was not marrying my wounding. Though there was a decent chance it would rip open his heart, ruining our marriage, he vowed to love the whole of me, in sickness and in health.

Every bit of old drama simply desires an empathetic, conscious witness, and my husband had provided that lovingly to me. Each of us longs to hold this kind of non-judgmental space for a loved one. This largeness of consciousness feels like freedom.

Now here's the rub. Here's the wisdom. The luminous gem. I do not have shame about the event.

The next day I knew that he'd handled it this way because he could see I had this storm brewing in me and it had to be let out. Instead of believing my shit, he just stared at me. I was and am so grateful for his wisdom. And for my growth.

Life can be like that. Think about when you're on the other end of a shit storm—as if you were on my husband's end. How will you respond? And if you are on the 'choose your weapon and fight me' side… how did that come to be? How can you learn from it? How can you bring forgiveness to your heart?

Don't be a voyeur in other people's dramas. Don't feed off of their struggles and sit higher to watch in judgment. Be willing to sit in your own shit and ask Shammah to burn it down.

In becoming whole I did not, as I expected, become impervious to needing others. Wholeness allows us to be fully aware of our need for our community, our family, our partners to be integral in our hu-maning.

Oh, yeah, baby: that is absolutely the time to make some shapes with the body.

be a warrior or a goddess
take your seat of righteousness
in chair pose
be an immovable mountain
then rest in your child-like nature
soar on an eagle's wings
allow the spine to move in six directions
and release the sweet elixir of the word made flesh
into your own hungry Self

the book of life has been written
into
your
very
bones

Crown Story

I was in my mid forties and struggling with memory issues.

I'd told myself maybe I had early Alzheimer's. I didn't feel I could learn new things. I was certain that, if I challenged myself, I would fail. (I did fail my yoga teacher training exam, not once, but twice. I was quick to place blame on my teachers; still cycling through victim mentality).

What happened to my good brain?

Perhaps raising children turned it to mush. That's the story I told myself for a bit. And, eventually, I said to my husband I was going to see a neurologist at Penn despite assurances that it's normal to have memory slips at my age.

At the specialist's office, I was asked, by an assistant, to draw a clock (the standard test) and I remember thinking 'this proves nothing'. Shortly after, a big-shot neurologist entered the room and asked me a few questions, then proclaimed: There's nothing wrong with you. You're a bored housewife.

I was furious. I felt helpless. And I had a few choice words.

So, I turned to my friend, Google, typing in: what holistic things can I do to help my brain?

Up popped a book called *How God Changes Your Brain* (Drs. Andrew B. Newberg and Mark Robert Waldman). One of its authors was a colleague of the neurologist I'd just seen. Classic, right?

I sent off a somewhat nasty email to the neurologist: you could have recommended your own colleague's book, suggested ginkgo biloba, for Christ's sake! Ultimately, I wrote thank you for pissing me off with your rude comment. I'll figure this out for myself. I'll let this light a fire under my own butt.

And I did. Up until this crisis of mental health, I'd been doing the physical postures of yoga for about six years, but had not meditated (one of the other eight limbs). The only people I knew at that time who were meditating were following more of a new age path or were utilizing visualization. I did not have even a basic understanding that nearly all mental disorders are rooted in early life, interpersonal mother-child context.

When we have hidden, unhealed trauma in the body-mind we cannot directly jump to more advanced practices. I see in the church that leaders often expect people to enter the silence of Centering Prayer (our version of silent contemplation). But it is extremely difficult to do this if those people are traumatized and have not been prepared with sufficient grounding and nervous system regulation through movement and breathing.

I went through the book, reading carefully, then began with a practice that utilized repetitive sound as well as moving the fingers.

Sa ta na ma. That shit was magic.

This was the first meditation I learned. Just repeating Sa Ta Na Ma aloud, then silently over and over, I lulled my anxious Self. I felt calmer, safer to remain inside when the difficult memories arose. Eventually, I advanced from sitting with a mantra to lying down in stillness and silence.

I cried every day for weeks as my body began to trust me to soften. Hours in our new hot tub, back in a dark, warm womb. Sliding underneath the bubbles to that place of no-thingness. The genesis of me. My suffering Self knew I had shown up in earnest. There would be no more self-abandonment. I had come in peace.

In a few weeks, my new mind was so dramatically healed that I knew this is what I would share with others. First, I balked—told God I wasn't ready, didn't have it mastered, needed more time. Blah blah blah. But when He breathed my lungs and instructed me with a simple: *"Go, you have my love. That is enough."* I found myself across from a dozen men in prison.

I knew this practice had the power to set us all free.

You can read everything by Eckhardt Tolle, and take in the *Untethered Soul* by Singer, and allow these concepts of awakening to entice you from the pages. You can read about white supremacy and systemic racism (which we white people all should), but not stop there—act, donate, humbly protest. Remember talk is cheap.

You can keep contemplating kenosis and what the mystics had to say about the dark night. You can cycle endlessly through blame and shame until your last breath. Or you can hop on your mat and practice collapsing old paradigms.

> *The dormant in you, which is the dormant in the Christ in you,*
> *is the one who will rise first.*

Better to brave the truth now.

May your world brighten. May vivid thinking replace stagnation. May the observer see through the illusion that there is a separate, controlling, lonely Self. May my words produce encouragement, never fear. Brain chemicals can flood us with a 'high' and these moments will change life forever because we will find ourselves more nurturing, peacekeepers. The once absent feminine aspects of Sophia wisdom will keep bringing to mind 'we' over 'me'. Gaze at one interpretation of Her on the book cover.

Therapy, in all its many forms from talk to somatic, and yoga are some of our tools. God is not a tool and neither are we 'tools' in the hands of a manipulating God. He called us friend, partner, bride, child; never were we inanimate. Once we make the primordial switch to never having been an object to being used or controlled by God, we halt making objects of our earth, one another, and our own bodies. We consciously decide to abandon the entire domination system we've been operating under.

ALL THE LOVE. ALL THE DAYS.

Together, we uncovered a universal truth: the Son comes in the now to save us from projecting the savior energy onto others, to save us from shame. When we bring our focus back to the inner child, to the expansion of the soul, we realize we've unearthed a new breed of human. We are participating in our own saving and renewal. I invited you to explore inside many of the recesses of my mind- thank you for taking this journey with me. I am honored to call you friend now.

Are we ready to be Kamikaze Yogis? I dream of the day we are a real community hashtagging our goofy pictures, encouraging one another.

It's what the Self ultimately desires: to be in this body, of this earth. Connecting heart to heart. Just one ordinary person to another, revealing an extraordinary God. I am wondering if the toxic lies about a judging Father have left our country's evangelicals seeking earthly power in the wake of disappointment that God's power never met them in their need.

I had no idea that to live in my comfort zone was slowly killing me from the inside. Sure, in many ways, before my awakening, life was simpler but predictable, far from enchanting and headed for disaster. If you don't explore the contents of the mind, you'll be left believing every thought. You'll be left assuming they are 'you'. And you'll be left having no idea where your power is.

*"God's not going to heal you apart from your participation.
He's got way more respect for us."*

WM. PAUL YOUNG, THE SHACK

Uncovering, then integrating the shadow, the unseen, untouched, unloved parts of ourselves is a Herculean task, but it is a deeply humbling journey that leads to ordinary as well as occasionally ecstatic union (like our mystics told us). I trust in my heart of hearts that, if it's true for me, it's true for everyone: simply keep going. I have found a universal pattern where discipline and submission to God overlap and create a third force: heaven on earth.

I tackled many fears while creating this book baby. If you've been called a heretic and preached at from the pulpit for not being a cookie-cutter Christian, there is space at the table now. If you are a Christ-follower afraid to break rank, know I see you and applaud you. Or maybe you are a yogi who left the faith behind? Each of us has a story that matters to God.

Mental healthcare in our country is extremely limited and is no match for the extent of suffering. We need more tools in our toolbox on a daily basis to recall our wholeness and bring us hope. We need to battle lethargy with routine and a reason.

Humanity's co-ascension in Christ is the whole point of the gospel—that's my take on Eph 2:5-6. Mystically speaking, we are already ascended into glory because He is our head, and we are His body. What if Abram was the man living in ignorance and separation before he was reborn in the spirit as Abraham, a new breed of human? Saul to Paul. Sarai to Sarah. Jacob to Israel. Simon to Peter. Each example someone who wrestled with God, with evil, with suffering, and with fellow man—each new name representing the covenant empowering a sacred mission. This is for humanity's benefit, not simply a personal dawning. He's drawing all people to himself. Yes, He's drawing *you* into a blessing of vitality—you need only to say yes to the adventure.

Many have not yet awakened to this truth. Will you be their clue?

Before we say farewell, I invite you to close your eyes, recalling a time when you felt really free, really powerful.

How does your body feel when you sit with this memory?

Author and minister, Lisa Bevere, recently did a powerful Instagram teaching on how lions must shift posture before they can roar.

Lions and Lionesses: may you arise in humility knowing your Lord is without rival. May you ask for a new name, even if it is just a private redeeming of one of your chakra demons. May your proclamation of your new identity release a change in the atmosphere. May you walk taller in a posture of assurance because it is sacred to be conscious of your divine nature. To see the world from your soul is to see everyone as already included in the Trinity, not a project, not lost.

This bodily knowing can replace the state of anxiety and depression with the tools in this book. May you come into direct contact with the divine therapist, and know that He is part of you, you are in Him, and the mind's divisions grow evermore dim from the heart's point of view. We were promised that the Comforter would explain what we need to know. May ancient texts which once lay flat on a page be inspirited to leap into your newly revived heart-mind.

I pushed through fear and doubt nearly every day for over two years of writing. I utilized my good, strong body to release them. Every day, I decided that the joy was in the giving, the creation of a thing. The Holy Spirit was loyal in fortifying me to execute Her will. May you be bold and open in receiving the gift of steadfast faith.

The chakra demons' masks hide the true face of Love. He is ascended into heaven and sits at the right hand of God the Father. We must confront those chakra demons in order for the power to birth ourselves as new humans. Like in the lyrics:, I found the heart of a lion in the belly of the beast. It's the heroine's journey… all the same universal message about bravery—and discovery—with Christian language.

One of my Easts pointed me back to embrace scripture—once I'd created some space inside of me.

The world needs your participaction. But you need your participaction most. You need to see yourself in three years. What are you doing? What's different about your life? You'll find, when you open your body, you literally breathe in the abundance of light. You, like Jesus, are distinct and unique. When you choose Him, He chooses you back. Jesus, the finite hu-man becomes the Christ because *we* are the witness to his arising. The lamb slain in the darkness of humanity's separation is miraculously transformed into a lion roaring an audacious gospel.

Come full circle: yes, you are the cracked vessel from which the divine, fragrant elixir pours. Yes, you must be smiling because you are such a phenomenon. Feeling an inexplicable sonder, you are filled with ambitions and worries. I hope you moved into a more permanent state of peace within a complicated earthly reality. Standing in your luminosity, bathe in the heavenliness of it all.

Now, this now, like no other *now* you breathed in before it, I pray you encounter a largeness of consciousness which makes space for the anger, the grief, the betrayal and the pain. On the other side you'll be enchanted by vibrant, inexplicable joy. That's because:

You are the one Jesus loves best, you new breed of hu-man.

EPILOGUE

I made you a special playlist on Spotify with my favorite songs under the book title. You can scan the QR code below to access it. These 25 songs bring John 9:37 to life "Jesus told us, 'you have seen Him, He is speaking with you.'"

"Come on down Daddy"
Love,
Anita

Connect with Anita Grace Brown

✉ kamikazeyogi2021@gmail.com

⬜ anitagracebrown2021

🐦 @anitagracebrown

SHAIA-SOPHIA
HOUSE

Shaia-Sophia House is a collaborative effort of
Alexander John Shaia and Nora Sophia's passion to
provide a creative home for fresh works from the
great traditions. We begin as a publishing house
with plans to expand soon into various mediums.

www.ShaiaSophiaHouse.com